THE HEALING POWERS OF VINEGAR

THE HEALING POWERS OF VINEGAR

A Complete Guide to Nature's Most Remarkable Remedy

CAL OREY

KENSINGTON BOOKS
http://www.kensingtonbooks.com

Heinz trademarks are owned by the H.J. Heinz Company and Heinz Information is used with permission.

KENSINGTON BOOKS are published by

Kensington Publishing Corp.
850 Third Avenue
New York, NY 10022

ISBN 1-57566-609-X

First Printing: October, 2000
10 9

Printed in the United States of America

CONTENTS

Foreword vii

PART 1 A Time for Vinegar

1. The Power of Vinegar 3
2. A Genesis of Sour Wine 11

PART 2 Apple Cider Vinegar

3. A Historical Testimony 19
4. Where Are the Secret Ingredients? 26
5. Why Is Apple Cider Vinegar So Healthy? 41

PART 3 Red Wine Vinegar

6. The Red Wine Vinegar Chronicle 57
7. The Old and New Healthful Ingredients 61
8. Tapping Into the French Paradox 68
9. Is Red Wine Vinegar Good for You? 74

PART 4 Other Natural Vinegars

10. Healthy Rice Vinegar 87
11. The Balsamic Vinegar Boom 92
12. Healing Herbal Vinegars 99

PART 5 Future Vinegar

13. Combining Vinegars and Garlic, Onions, and Olive Oil 109
14. Vinegarmania: Hope or Hype? 121

PART 6 Vinegar Remedies

15. Therapeutic Uses 135
16. Vinegar Is Not for Everyone: Some Sour Views 150

PART 7 Vinegar Recipes 153

PART 8 Vinegar Resources 245

Notes 256

Foreword

You have always known that vinegar tasted great on your french fries, and dressed up your salad and made your glassware sparkle, but now you will learn of the many medicinal uses of this magic liquid. For 10,000 years vinegar has been revered all around the world. In America it has been made from fruits and grains, the same way for over 200 years.

Vinegar has been a trusted home remedy that your mother, your grandmother, and their grandmothers have known. It literally can be used from head to toe. Scalp problems such as dandruff, athlete's foot, yeast infections, even headaches, are no match for this remedy. It can also be used as a cosmetic, to help protect and beautify your skin.

Some forms of vinegar are a virtual storehouse of important vitamins, over a dozen minerals, essential amino acids, and several enzymes, as well as beta-carotene. Cooking with vinegar is truly a delightful experience.

In *The Healing Power of Vinegar,* Cal Orey will reveal to you the secrets of red wine vinegar, apple cider vinegar, and other natural vinegars as well as combining them with other time-honored remedies.

Even where the best place to buy the stuff. Come along with us through the sweetness of this sour product.

—Dr. Earl Mindell, author of *The Vitamin Bible for the 21st Century* and *Dr. Earl Mindell's Herb Bible*

PART 1

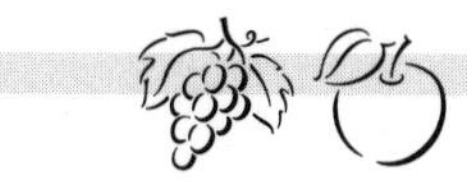

A TIME FOR VINEGAR

CHAPTER

1

The Power of Vinegar

Vinegar, the son of wine.

—Babylonian Talmud: Baba Metzia[1]

Angelo Salcia* is a 91-year-old man who uses his Italian family's old-fashioned remedies for good health. Every day he takes one tablespoon of raw, unfiltered apple cider vinegar in a glass of warm water. After years of using this apple cider vinegar "cocktail," this senior remains active in body and spirit. He vows the golden liquid helps keep his blood thin and prevents arthritis.

For Theresa Gariddo,* a woman with strong Basque roots, red wine vinegar is a handed down folk remedy is well worth holding onto. At 35, she is a dental office manager in San Francisco, California, wife, and mom. When her fun-loving toddler, Eric, bumped his head on a doorframe at her parent's house, vinegar came to the rescue. "My mom took a quarter and pushed it against the welt," she recalls. "Right after, we used red wine vinegar and salt. It takes away the inflammation and makes it heal faster, so they say." And it did.

Max Lombari,* aged 67, believes that the vinegar in his diet is one

*Some names of individuals have been changed to protect their privacy.

reason why he has no major health problems. As a regular customer at Salvatore's Continental Restaurant of San Carlos, California, Max always orders red wine vinegar on the side to put on his pasta salad. "He told me vinegar is good for your health," says the chef, Sal Campagna, a vinegar connoisseur who makes his own flavorful vinegar.

For these and countless other people with roots in the old Mediterranean world, the healing powers of vinegar are well known. These people use vinegar not only as a versatile home remedy but also as an integral part of the renowned Mediterranean diet, where it provides an additional health boost by teaming up with fruits, vegetables, grains, and olive oil.

If you haven't heard by now, listen up. Your health may depend on it. Chances are, you already have two great folk remedies in your kitchen cupboards. It's time to start using them more.

Medical doctors and even scientists are now saying just what folk herbalists in Europe have been saying for years, that *both* apple cider vinegar and red wine vinegar may have a host of amazing healing powers.

I remember as a teenager my mother made sure that I ate my "good for you" dinner. She used both apple cider vinegar and red wine vinegar in her dishes. On Sunday nights I enjoyed eating a fresh cucumber salad: sliced cucumbers, tomatoes, and onions smothered in red wine vinegar. And for dessert, a homemade apple pie was our treat. Real apples were always used for their wholesome goodness and apple cider vinegar for that extra tang. Well, it turns out Mom knew best.

Today, we know even more about the natural goodness behind these two vinegars. Both apple cider vinegar and red wine vinegar are good folk medicine. And this healthful duo promises to be a major home remedy in the new millennium, when alternative medicine will be widespread.

Health Fact!

A survey published in *The Journal of the American Medical Association* shows that Americans paid more office visits to alternative medicine practitioners than to primary care physicians.[2]

Medical researchers believe some known trace elements and even the new health-promoting "nutraceuticals" (nutrient supplements that act like pharmaceuticals which are currently being researched for their potential to treat cancer and heart disease) may be in apple cider vinegar and red wine vinegar.

In addition, foods that are nutritious and prevent diseases are called "functional foods," according to the American Dietetic Association. Scientists have linked functional foods with the prevention or treatment of cancer, diabetes, and heart disease. And studies are ongoing.

The Apple and the Grape Yield Two Powerful Vinegars

Apple cider vinegar has been touted by vinegar gurus as one of nature's most healthful foods, especially if made from fresh, organically grown apples, then allowed to age. And now, red wine vinegar, the ignored condiment, may be its new sidekick, thanks to the grape known as "the vine healer."

People from all walks of life—as well as some vinegar pioneers and contemporary medical experts—believe apple-rich apple cider vinegar aids digestion, helps maintain weight, and keeps blood pressure down. Apple cider vinegar is also known to relieve congestion and maintain healthy skin.

One of the earliest doctors to praise apple cider vinegar was D. C. Jarvis, M.D. Dr. Jarvis strongly recommends its use in his book *Folk Medicine: A New England Almanac of Natural Health Care from a Noted Vermont Country Doctor*, a book that promotes alternative medicine. It's the potassium content, says Jarvis, that makes apple cider vinegar work. "It is so essential to the life of every living thing that without it there would be no life."[3]

Potassium Plus in Apple Cider Vinegar

It's unanimous. As you learn more about apple cider vinegar, you'll continue to hear about the wonders of its high potassium content. Potassium in apple cider vinegar promotes cell, tissue, and organism growth.

In addition to potassium, apple cider vinegar contains these and other health boosters:

Enzymes: chemical substances your body produces to help boost chemical reactions in your body.

Calcium: necessary for transmitting nerve impulses, regulating muscle contraction, and maintaining healthy bones.

Iron: an essential mineral which is important for your blood.

Magnesium: a mineral which has many beneficial effects on you body, most important its impact on heart health.

Two of America's popular antiaging health authorities, Dr. Paul Bragg and Dr. Patricia Bragg, spread the good word about potassium-rich apple cider vinegar's health benefits, too. This health-minded team gives credit to apple cider vinegar as being one of the best aids to health and long life known to mankind. They give kudos to its natural substance produced by powerful enzymes—living chemicals.[4]

And now, New Age doctors claim red grapes yield another amazing vinegar. *Red wine vinegar*, claim medical experts, contains healthful nutrients that are part of the "neutraceutical revolution," too. While it's apples that make apple cider vinegar what it is, it is the grape that may be the core of red wine vinegar's nutrients.

For example, one of the nation's leading authorities in preventive, nutritional, and environmental medicine, Allan Magaziner, D.O., founder and director of the Magaziner Center for Wellness and Anti-Aging Medicine in Cherry Hill, New Jersey, says red wine vinegar may have some disease-fighting antioxidant vitamins which are not listed on its label—and yet can be beneficial to our health and well-being.

Andrew Waterhouse, Ph.D., a wine chemist at the University of California at Davis agrees. Like in wine, red wine vinegar may contain a "new class" of antioxidants or polyphenolics—quercetin, catchechins, tannins—which may lower the risk of heart disease and cancer.

Both vinegars have been noted for their folklore remedies in ancient history to modern times, and have gained the respect of countless people, past and present. Before I provide a guide to the health virtues of vinegar, here's what you need to know.

Polyphenols in Red Wine Vinegar

Like apple cider vinegar, red wine vinegar contains polyphenols, naturally occurring compounds that act as powerful antioxidants (enzymes that protect your body by trapping the free-radical molecules and getting rid of them before damage occurs).

Science continues to find new "cutting edge" health-promoting nutrients in grapes and red wine, and these may be in red wine vinegar:

Catechin: a flavonoid believed to prevent cancer.

Flavonoids: antioxidants which belong to the phytochemical family. They are the substances found in fruit and vegetables that give them their colors and flavors.

Quercetin: belongs to the class of nutrients known as bioflavonoids which provides allergy relief and has been shown to protect from stomach disorders.

Resveratrol: a compound which may have anticancer properties; and may have substances which can also protect against heart disease.

Vinegar Basics 101

Vinegar is one of the oldest fermented food products known to man—except for wine and perhaps certain foods made from milk. The word "vinegar" comes from the French *vin aigre* which means "sour wine," a definition that is a no-brainer to anyone who has left a bottle of Chardonnay exposed to the air too long. And someone did just that about 10,000 years ago.

So what exactly is vinegar, anyhow? Simply put, when air is exposed to a fermented liquid, like wine or ale, bacterial activity occurs. This process helps combine oxygen with the alcohol. The end result: acetic acid or sour vinegar.

Vinegar: 1. an impure dilute solution of acetic acid obtained by fermentation beyond alcohol stage and used as a condiment and preservative. 2. Sourness of speech or mood; ill temper. 3. Liveliness and enthusiasm; vim.

—*The American Heritage Dictionary*

Vinegar can be made from any fruit, such as apples or grapes, or any material containing sugar. The following kinds of vinegar are categorized according to material from which they are made and method of production.

VINEGAR POTPOURRI

Kind	Materials Made From	Method of Making
Apple cider vinegar	Apples, apple juice	Twofold fermentation
Wine vinegar	Grapes, peaches, and berries	Twofold fermentation
Malt vinegar	Barley malt or other cereals where starch has been converted into maltose	Twofold fermentation
Sugar vinegar	Solutions of sugar, syrup, or molasses	Twofold fermentation
Spirit or distilled vinegar	Alcohol which comes from whole grain products	Acetic fermentation of dilute distilled alcohol

Source: The Vinegar Institute.

High-tech manufacturing companies speed up the vinegar-making process. Their method is to circulate fermented liquid through large vats, incorporating lots of air and quickly producing a product. Better-quality vinegars, however, are often left unfiltered and unpasteurized, in which case the bacteria or "mother" will form at the top.

Mother or "mother-of-vinegar" is a term used to describe the excess liquid which accumulates on top of cider or other juice, which turns them into the most nutritious vinegars for health. As the fermentation progresses, mother forms a floating clump or filmy substance, like a coffee latte with the foam on top. Mother, the latte-like foam, is a living mixture of "good" bacteria and enzymes.

All-Natural Orleans Process

The slower the conversion from wine to vinegar, the better the vinegar will be. If you're looking for good vinegar, you want one that's been made using the traditional, all-natural Orleans process, which takes weeks, not hours, to make vinegar. Early vinegar experts fine-tuned this method during the Middle Ages in Orleans, France.[5]

The best vinegars are made from whole apples ground into pulp, cold-pressed to extract the cider, fermented in wooden barrels, and aged for at least six months. Organic cider vinegars are available at health-food stores and usually unfiltered. Other kinds are made from apple cores and peelings, then quickly processed. Some companies, such as Heinz, follow the traditional process of pressing whole apples for their juice.

Naturally Organic

Organic vinegars are made from fruits and grains that are not sprayed with chemical insecticides or pesticides. Natural types of repellents and fertilizers without chemical pesticides and fewer sulfites (a food additive) are used instead. Also the vinegars are free of chemicals or additives. In addition, natural vinegars are free of artificial colorings, flavorings, dyes, and preservatives.

Though the acidity and nutrient content of vinegars may vary, legal standards in America require vinegar to be at least 4 percent acidity, or 4 grams of acetic acid per 100 cubic centimeters. Most are 5 percent acidity. The acidity is defined by the word "grain," which refers to the amount of water dilution. For instance, a 40-grain vinegar is 4 percent acetic acid.[6]

Despite vinegar's acidity strength, health experts are now discovering what the old country folks knew all along: both apple cider vinegar and red wine vinegar have amazing healing powers.

Important Healing Hints to Remember

New evidence shows that *both* apple cider and red wine vinegars—which are made from whole apples and red grapes—may help you to:

✓ Fight fat.
✓ Enhance your immune system.
✓ Lower blood pressure.
✓ Lower risk of heart disease.
✓ Prevent cancer.
✓ Slow the aging process.

In this book, I will show you how using both vinegars can be one of the best things you do for yourself—and your health. But note, many people will not want to reap the benefits of vinegar by drinking the healthy brew solo. While vinegar is great for salad, it also is a great seasoning for many foods. Vinegar has a vast number of uses in cooking, and I've included more than 100 recipes to help heal your body, mind, and spirit.

But first, let's go way, way back into the past. Take a close-up look at why and how vinegar is one of the world's first—and most prized—natural medicines.

CHAPTER

2

A Genesis of Sour Wine

Pour vinegar and oil into the same cruse and thou wilt say that, as foes, they keep asunder.
—Aeschylus, *Agamemnon* (458 B.C.)[1]

As early as 400 B.C., Hippocrates used vinegar to treat his patients. In the era of the Romans and Egyptians, there were many potent vinegars on meal tables. During the nineteenth century, vinegar was used as a healing dressing, and in the twentieth century, people drank vinegar cocktails of all kinds.

Today, nutritionists and researchers around the world continue to utilize other powerful uses of this universal liquid. And history shows that people of yesteryear took advantage not only of the internal benefits of vinegar, but of its external virtues as well.

Vinegar's great power is timeless. The earliest historical record of vinegar may be the Babylonians. In 5,000 B.C. they made vinegar as an end product of a wine from the date palm. Since that time, vinegar has been used as a food preservative, a medicinal agent, an antibiotic, and even as a household cleaner. Then and now it's known for its "good" antimicrobial properties—it kills "bad" microorganisms.

Hippocrates, known as "the father of medicine," treated his patients with vinegar as an antibiotic. It was one of our first medicines. Hippocrates used vinegar to treat a variety of illnesses. For instance, he told his patients that oxymel (a honey and vinegar combination) was a good remedy for getting rid of phlegm and breathing easy. It is believed that strong acid, such as in the honey and vinegar, helps to clear up congestion.[2]

Hippocrates also prescribed this potent honey-vinegar combo for other ailments. Not only was oxymel to aid in regularity, but it also treated respiratory disorders such as peripneumonia and pleurisy, too. Vinegar was used to treat inflammations and swellings and even burns. Also, the ancient medicine man used vinegar for disinfecting ulcerations.[3]

Vinegar is mentioned eight times in the Bible: four times in the Old Testament and four in the New Testament. In fact, there is even a Vinegar Bible. In the sixteenth century the Clarendon Press in Oxford, England, typeset the word "vinegar" instead of "vineyard" in the top-of-the-page running headline of the twenty-second chapter of Luke. And soon, the edition was coined the "Vinegar Bible."[4]

Since Biblical times, vinegar, known as "the poor man's wine," has played a major role in the lives of both the rich, such as in royalty, and in the poor. Laborers, for instance, would add a splash of wine vinegar to water, perhaps with a pinch of salt. This ancient version of an energizing drink was teamed with bread to help people persevere as they

The Royal Power of Vinegar

Remember Cleopatra, the legendary Queen of Egypt? The strong-willed African woman led her husband, Mark Antony, into an ironic, no-win wager. She put her vinegar smarts to work. According to Pliny, a Roman scholar, the savvy queen claimed that she could eat one meal which would cost a million sisteries (an old Roman coin). The bet seemed absurd, since one human can only consume so much at one sitting, right? Not exactly.

The queen simply dropped a million sisteries' worth of pearls into a glass of vinegar. Meanwhile, the "meal" was put aside while food preparations were made. At mealtime, the queen just swallowed the dissolved pearls. Thanks to her vinegar knowledge—she knew the acidic strength of sour wine—the "liquid meal" was not only an expensive one, but a sure-fire way to win the bet.

worked under the hot sun. Even in the eighteenth and nineteenth centuries, this age-old vinegar tradition was used by laborers. For example, a fruit-flavored vinegar known as "shurbs" or "switches" was used by workers during harvesting.[5]

During the Middle Ages, vinegar made its mark, too. Four robbers in the French town of Marseilles preyed upon the homes and belongings left behind by the people who fell victim to the bubonic plague, or "Black Death" of Europe. Eventually they were caught and brought before French judges, who wondered how these four thieves had protected themselves from the deadly plague while looting plague-ridden possessions.

The legend is that the four thieves bargained and exchanged the famous Four Thieves Vinegar formula for their freedom, explaining that they washed themselves with the infection-fighting liquid every few hours. Upon learning about these immunity-boosting qualities, the formula was used by priests and doctors who treated the ill.

No one seems to know who wrote the formula, which differs from recipe to recipe, but it is basically the same and it works in various ways. It can be used to disinfect sick rooms. If diluted with water, it can be used as a body wash. Taken by the teaspoonful (consult with your doctor for the safe amount), it can be used as a preventive measure to stave off viral infections, such as the flu.

Therapeutic Formula of the Four Thieves

Basic ingredients: Combine 3 quarts apple cider vinegar; 3 tablespoons *each* of rosemary, lavender, sage, mint, rue, and plantain; and 6 cloves of garlic. Let it sit in a covered container for at least 24 hours.

In the American Civil War, vinegar is believed to have prevented scurvy—the disease caused by a vitamin C deficiency. It was also used as a disinfectant and healing agent to treat wounds in both the American Civil War and World War I.[6]

OTHER PAST MEDICAL USES OF VINEGAR

Historical Vinegar User	Method	Ailment
Assyrian tablets[7]	Vinegar	For ear diseases
Ancient Persian Physicians[8]	Mixture of lime juice, the sour juice of certain fruits, and vinegar	To prevent fat accumulation in the body
Greek, Roman, and Asian doctors[9]	Vinegar	Aiding digestion, preventing scurvy, lowering bile levels
Spartianus, historian[10]	Mixture of vinegar and water	Helped soldiers survive rigors of battle
Medieval people[11]	Herbal vinegar with lavender and rosemary	Unease of stomach and brain
Galen, doctor in the second century A.D.[12]	Honey and vinegar	Coughs
B. Boyles, fellow of Royal Society of London[13]	Vinegar	Used as a gargle
Genteel people of the 17th/18th centuries[14]	Vinegar-soaked sponges	To ward off the noxious odors of raw sewage and garbage
Hippocrates[15]	Vinegar, honey, and pepper	Feminine disorders
Egyptians[16]	Vinegar	Mushroom poisoning, worms in the ears, bleeding wounds, severe loss of appetite, and gangrene
Theophrastus, a Greek[17]	Mixture of vinegar with pepper	Revives a victim of suffocation

TWENTIETH-CENTURY VINEGAR MILESTONES

Year	What Happened	What It Did
1909	Dr. Jarvis began studying herbal medicines and folk remedies after he began practicing medicine.	Helped treat people with ACV for a variety of ailments.
1912	Dr. Alexis Carrel began an experiment that successfully kept the cells of an embryo chicken heart alive for 30 years.	Showed the importance of ACV in health and longevity.
1958	*Folk Medicine: A Vermont Doctor's Guide to Good Health* was published.	Chronicled the ACV remedies Dr. D.C. Jarvis studied to treat many diseases.
1968	On January 17, the Vinegar Institute began.	Helped vinegar producers to protect their rights.
1973	Marcella Hazan, a cooking teacher and author, introduced America to balsamic vinegar from the provinces of Modena and Reggio Emilia.[18]	
1990s	The Braggs provided self-help books: such as *Apple Cider Vinegar: Miracle Health System*	Helped teach people to live healthier lives.
1999	On June 4, in Roslyn, South Dakota, the international Vinegar Museum was opened.	It will inform you about the wonderful power of vinegar.

IMPORTANT HEALING HINTS TO REMEMBER

As you can see, versatile vinegar has been praised for centuries—in the United States and around the world—as a healing medicine. Vinegar devotees, past and present, believe that vinegar—both ACV and RWV—can fight disease and add years to your life by:

- ✓ Acting as a safe and effective natural preservative in food.
- ✓ Fighting deadly food bacteria.
- ✓ Aiding in digestion.
- ✓ Preventing infection.
- ✓ Enhancing immune system function.
- ✓ Fighting viruses.

No doubt, vinegar back then had a wide variety of powerful health benefits. And it's managed to hold up to its good name. Now it's time to get the lowdown on one of the nation's most popular kinds of vinegar—apple cider vinegar—then . . . and now.

PART 2

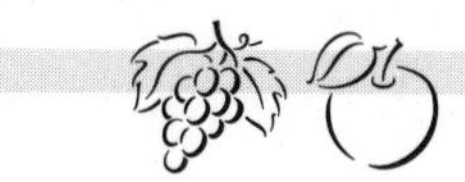

Apple Cider Vinegar

CHAPTER

3

A Historical Testimony

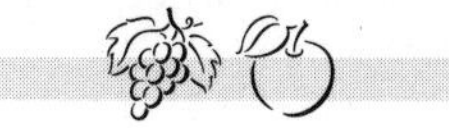

Sour makes sweet happen.

—The Vinegar Man[1]

Paul Bragg reminisces about his father in his book *Apple Cider Vinegar: Miracle Health System.* He recalls his early youth when he enjoyed "robust health" on an apple farm. He wrote, "I was a great apple eater. Each year my father made natural Apple cider vinegar and stored it in wooden barrels. On our table we used this natural Apple cider vinegar and our large family loved it."[2]

Bragg was impressed by his hardworking father. Often he would watch him add apple cider vinegar to the feed and water of sick farm animals and watched it restore health to cattle, horses, sheep, dogs, and cats. The apple cider vinegar worked like a magical potion. Because the farm family lived out in the country, they turned to self-health remedies like vinegar.[3]

The apple cider vinegar advocate remembers his father working long hours during harvest time. His father would be up before dawn and work without rest until late at night. Bragg observed him come into the kitchen and fix a honey and apple cider vinegar cocktail. "I would say, 'Father, why do you drink vinegar, honey and water?' And father would reply, 'Son, farm work is long hard work, it can produce chronic fatigue in the body.'" Bragg learned about a powerful ingredient in that drink that renewed his father's vitality and relieved him of fatigue and stiffness. That ingredient was potassium, which along with healthful enzymes, minerals, and trace elements, are all found in apple cider vinegar.[4]

Apple cider vinegar gurus of the 1900s such as Dr. Paul C. Bragg and Dr. Patricia Bragg will not be forgotten. This father-and-daughter health-minded team believe apple cider vinegar has internal and external benefits which include: helping to control and normalize weight, improve digestion, promote a youthful, healthy body, and even prevent dandruff.

Paul and Patricia Bragg: ACV Pioneers

Paul Bragg: World Health Crusader. Bragg, N.D., Ph.D., life extension specialist, originated, named, and opened the first "Health Food Store" in America. He introduced juice therapy in America by bringing the first hand-operated vegetable-fruit juicer from Germany. He was the first to introduce and distribute honey nationwide. He inspired millions to "go organic" in their gardening.
Patricia Bragg: Paul Bragg's daughter, N.D., Ph.D., a Doctor of Naturopathy, and health and fitness expert, carries on the family name. She lectures on health via radio and TV.

Source: Live Food Products: C. S. Lewis & Co. Publicists.

THE VERMONT COUNTRY DOCTOR

These two vinegar advocates shared the same path that great folk medicine doctor D. C. Jarvis traveled, too. This family doctor noticed that many of his patients—down-to-earth country people—used folk remedies to prevent and treat most illnesses.

Dr. Jarvis offers many uses for apple cider vinegar. Apple cider vinegar is used for many ailments, from poison ivy, burns (including sunburn), varicose veins, impetigo, and bacterial infections, to more serious problems—such as high blood pressure in one of his patients. (See Chapter 15: "Therapeutic Uses.")

Acid-Alkaline = Better Blood: A Vermont woman showed a whopping blood pressure reading of nearly 300 when it was taken at a clinic, reports Dr. Jarvis. "However, by controlling the alkalinity of her blood in the manner taught by Vermont folk medicine, she was able to live to the age of 84 years," he says. How? In a nutshell: She upped her daily intake of acid in organic form. That can be in the form of apples or two teaspoons of apple cider vinegar in a glass of water.[5]

A high-protein, high-fat diet increases the alkalinity in the blood, causing it to thicken as in this Vermont patient. It is believed by Dr. Jarvis that apple cider vinegar affects the acid-alkali balance. It thins the blood, which may help lower blood pressure and improve blood circulation.

Today, the American diet high in meat and lower in alkalizing fruits and vegetables leaves an acid residue in the body. The acid residue, in turn, imbalances our biochemistry or pH blood levels in a direction where we are out of acid-alkaline balance. And that can lead to high blood pressure and other heart ailments, say vinegar experts.

"Thus, it is necessary for you to eat as much vegetables as possible to prevent acidity in your body fluid, which may result from taking too much animal protein," reports Togo Kuroiwa in his book *Rice Vinegar: An Oriental Home Remedy.*[6] The organic acids found in fruits, vegetables, and apple cider vinegar provide the body with important minerals such as potassium, calcium, sodium, and magnesium. These and other minerals form compounds in the body that turn acid body fluids alkaline. Because of this, they are called alkalizing minerals, and the food that supply them—such as apple cider vinegar—are called alkalizing foods. Animal proteins and other acidifying foods cause the body fluids to be more acid, which favors bacterial growth and leads to disease. That's why to stay healthy, our bodies need a constant fresh supply of the alkalizing minerals that are found in fruits, vegetables, and apple cider vinegar.

Food Poison Prevention. Another one of the Vermont doctor's patients experienced the quick healing power of apple cider vinegar. At a Shriner's summer picnic in Vermont, lobster salad was the main course. The salad was spoiled and nineteen people suffered the consequences: food poisoning. One of the diners had taken preventive measures. Dr. Jarvis advised him whenever there was any chance that food might be spoiled, use apple cider vinegar. "At the onset of dinner he poured a generous amount into his glass of water. It happened that he was particularly fond of lobster salad and he had two extra helpings. Whereas many of his table companions suffered bad effects from the spoiled lobster, the apple cider vinegar had so sterilized it in his digestive tract that nothing disagreeable happened to him."[7]

Lameness Rx. One day a farmer at Dr. Jarvis's office reported his bothersome arthritis. He told the doctor that before taking 10 teaspoonfuls of apple cider vinegar in a glass of water with each meal, he had lameness in all the joints of his body. The first day after he started taking apple cider vinegar, he reported his lameness was 20 percent better. The second day he said he was 50 percent better. By the end of a month 75 percent improvement. Not only did the lameness clear up, but so did the pain.[8]

Dr. Carrel's Famous Longevity Experiment

Dr. Alexis Carrel, the New York City doctor back in 1912, administered apple cider vinegar daily to the cells of an embryo chicken heart. That was to ensure that it got a full quota of potassium. The normal life span of a chicken is 7½ to 8 years. Amazingly, Dr. Carrel kept the chicken heart alive and healthy for over three decades—thanks to potassium.

"Dr. Carrel definitely proved to the entire world that the body has a seed of eternal life that man kills himself by wrong habits of eating and living," the Braggs report. The conclusion: Apple cider vinegar is vital to good health and longevity. The question is, can it apply to human beings, too?[9]

Contemporary Doctors: The ACV Late Bloomers

"Do as I do—drink vinegar," said best-selling author Julian Whitaker, M.D., who has practiced medicine for over 20 years at the Whitaker Wellness Institute in Newport Beach, California. He is the author of *Reversing Hypertension: A Vital New Program to Prevent, Treat, and Reduce High Blood Pressure* (Warner Books, 2000) and other health books about the prevention of diabetes and heart disease. Dr. Whitaker admitted in May 1997 that for a few months he'd been drinking a glass of warm water with a teaspoon each of raw honey and apple cider vinegar once a day. "I'm not ready to commit to it as a ritual but there's enough anecdotal evidence for me to add it my daily routine."[10]

He is hardly alone. John, a 76-year-old man, had a variety of stomach woes all his life, reports Dr. Whitaker. "After countless GI workups, most recently a series of tests costing $2,000, he was told by his doctor that they could find nothing to explain these problems and recommended he take Zantac every day." But John took an alternative route. For one week he drank one teaspoon of raw, unfiltered, organic apple cider vinegar and one teaspoon of raw honey in warm water once a day. Afterward, his heartburn and stomach problems were no longer a problem.[11]

Dr. Whitaker recalls another man who gives a lot of credit to his "vinegar cocktails" which help remedy angina pain. At 66, Bob was being treated for heart disease. He mixed a shot glass of vinegar with molasses and grapefruit juice and downed it twice a day. "Of course," says Dr. Whitaker, "he was pursuing several other therapies for his chest pain at the same time, but he feels that the vinegar had a decided effect."[12]

Adds Dr. Whitaker: "This is pretty strong testimony for an unglamorous and inexpensive product like vinegar, but stories like this abound. Although it has little mention in the medical literature, apple cider vinegar has a solid and respected place in folk medicine."[13]

Perhaps its best known application is for indigestion, as John experienced so dramatically. Other conditions vinegar reportedly improves include arthritis, leg cramps, swimmer's ear (rinse with equal parts vinegar and water), urinary problems, and excess weight. When applied topically, it can relieve athlete's foot and dandruff, and it makes a good hair rinse, as thousands will attest.[14]

"Daily I drink two ounces of ACV because it's a great source of potassium, good for blood pressure and muscles since I run/walk every day," says Jan McBarron, M.D., a Columbus, Georgia, weight-loss specialist. Dr. McBarron lost 65 pounds—and she's kept it off for over 10 years. She also believes apple cider vinegar helps digestion and aids in staying regular.

You Can't Argue with Success

Plenty of people have reaped the health benefits of apple cider vinegar. Take a look at these success stories:

Longevity Booster. My dear friend Valerie Smith,* a musician who lives in Redwood City, California, believes apple cider vinegar is healthful. At 87, she believes in home remedies for good health. No unnatural drugs for her.

She recalls, "As a child I would daily drink apple cider vinegar straight from its container. I liked the tart taste." Today this octogenarian continues to use vinegar and remains mentally and physically energized. She still drives, dines, and attends the opera. Just one more of Mother Nature's miracles.

A Healthier Life. Bonnie Raley,* 52, has been using (and selling) apple cider vinegar with herbs (see Chapter 12: "Healing Herbal Vinegars") for 2½ years. "I have found that I have fewer colds, and if I do seem to be catching a cold, I can fight them off much better than before. I also have no more pain and stiffness in my ankles. I used to awaken with such stiffness that I had pain for several minutes of walking. I no longer have any pain or stiffness.

"My husband and I began taking it after our daughter was able to get her blood sugar in control after just 2 weeks. We have been so pleased with our level of energy and the way our bodies have been able to fight off colds and other viruses that other people seem to have.

"I also am going through menopause. I was having periods during the night in which I experienced 'hot flashes.' I no longer have this problem, however, it does recur if I forget to take the product for more than three or four days."

Digestion Protection. For 20 years Pat Gilmore,* 62, a psychologist in Burlingame, California, has turned to apple cider vinegar as an antibacteria protectant before going to a pot luck dinner. "I have no control over who puts what into what food or how clean their hands were. I want to eat their food—I don't want to be all picky and weird. So about a half hour before I go, I just take a tablespoon of vinegar and put it in a glass of cool water and drink it."

Apple Cider Vinegar Is Timeless

In short, apple cider vinegar was healthy in the twentieth century and is healthy in the twenty-first century, too. While its uses are plentiful—both inside and outside your body—its healing powers are due to its healthful ingredients. And now, research reveals more about apple cider vinegar nutrients (which may be missing from our daily food intake) more than ever before.

Important Healing Hints to Remember

- ✓ Potassium in apple cider vinegar may renew vitality and relieve fatigue.
- ✓ Apple cider vinegar has external and internal benefits—from dandruff to digestion.
- ✓ Apple cider vinegar may help lameness and heartburn.
- ✓ Apple cider vinegar may boost your immune system and add years to your life.

CHAPTER

4

Where Are the Secret Ingredients?

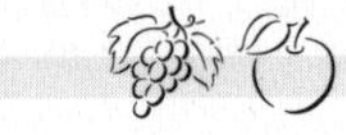

Natural apple cider vinegar
can really be called
one of nature's most perfect foods.[1]

—Drs. Bragg

At the dawn of the new millennium, after distilled white vinegar, apple cider vinegar is America's favorite. As far as vinegars go, it is still number one for both internal and external use.

People believe that apple cider vinegar, which is found in most of our homes, stores, and restaurants—and costs just pennies—can stave off arthritis, fight body fat, regulate blood pressure, and even maintain healthy bones. Sound silly? It's not, according to medical experts who believe in the power of home remedies.

The problem is, mainstream nutritionists, doctors, and apple cider vinegar makers play down the good-for-you nutrients in this liquid "cure-all." Even the vinegar trade associations will not link themselves to any health or nutritional claims. As for alternative health experts, even though they aren't exactly sure what accounts for vinegar's health benefits—owing to a lack of conclusive scientific data—they do agree that there is an enormous amount of anecdotal evidence of its healing powers. Here's what I discovered:

When you look at apple cider vinegar's product label, it appears to be a dieter's dream: no calories, fat, or sodium, right? But where are the potent nutrients, I pondered.

Nutrition Facts
Serving Size 1 Tablespoon (14)
Amount per serving

Calories 0

Calories from fat 0

Total Fat 0 g

Sodium 0 mg

Total Carbohydrate 0

Sugars 0 g

(*Source:* Eden Organic Apple Cider Vinegar.)

Dazed and confused, I went straight to the vinegar makers, and obtained a nutritional breakdown of the golden liquid. The nutrition facts seem to be a bit different, and the measurements a bit bigger.

More Apple Cider Vinegar, Anyone?

100 grams (three-and-one-half ounces) contains:
95% water
14 calories
0 protein
0 dietary fiber
0 fat
5 grams of carbohydrates
6 milligrams of calcium
9 milligrams of phosphorus
0.6 milligrams of iron
1 milligram of sodium
100 milligrams of potassium
22 milligrams of magnesium
0.04 milligrams of copper[2]

Apparently, more cider equals more nutrients. One cup contains:
98% water
34 calories
A trace of protein
0 fat

14.2 grams of carbohydrate
14 milligrams of calcium
22 milligrams of phosphorus
1.4 milligrams of iron
2 milligrams of sodium
240 milligrams of potassium[3]

People who have written about vinegar claim that apple cider vinegar contains more than thirty important nutrients, a dozen minerals, over half a dozen vitamins and essential acids, several enzymes, and pectin. The bottom line is that more research will be needed before more doctors—conventional and holistic alike—truly understand what accounts for vinegar's healing powers.

Quality Counts

Not all vinegar is nutritionally equal, natural, organic apple cider vinegar and made using the slow Orleans method. Some producers speed up the process so that vinegar can be bottled within three days.

"For medicinal purposes the apple cider vinegar should be made from the crushed whole apples," says Dr. Jarvis. "Following the line of changes when the whole apple is crushed to make apple cider vinegar," adds Dr. Jarvis, "it is found that the healthful properties in the original apple are passed down to the apple cider vinegar."[4]

The fact is, the best cider vinegars are made from whole apples ground into pulp, cold-pressed to extract the cider, fermented in wooden barrels, and aged for at least six months for rich full flavor. This is the ideal way.

Apple cider vinegar contains the same important nutrients as apples—pectin, beta-carotene, and potassium—plus it contains enzymes and amino acids which are formed during the fermentation process.

"Vinegar possesses the same essential nutrients as the ingredients originally used to make it, but gains nutrients during the fermentation process, notably enzymes and amino acids. Many believe it is the natural fermentation process which endows the final product with its diverse healing properties," explains co-author Earl L. Mindell in his book *Amazing Apple Cider Vinegar* (Keats Publishing, February 1, 1997).

Apple Nutrition

One apple contains 100 calories, mainly from carbohydrate; 2 grams of fiber; 10 mg vitamin C; 150 IUs vitamin A; modest amounts of B vitamins—B_1, B_2, B_3, B_6, and biotin; 159 mg of potassium; over 15 mg each of calcium, magnesium, and phosphorus; about 0.5 mg of iron; traces of maganese, copper, selenium, and zinc; some vitamin E (mostly in the seeds).[5]

(*Source: Staying Healthy with Nutrition: The Complete Guide to Diet and Nutritional Medicine*, Elson Haas, M.D., Celestial Arts, 1992.)

An Apple a Day Means Fewer Doctors to Pay

Eighty percent of the fiber found in an apple is soluble fiber—or pectin, which may be of help in lowering blood cholesterol levels. Also, apples are a good source of potassium, which helps provide protection against strokes. And like most other fruits, they're also lower in sodium (for better blood pressure), calories (for staying slim), and fat (for lower cholesterol).

Research suggests naturally occurring chemicals found in apples, called flavonoids, may reduce the risk of heart disease and inhibit the development of certain cancers, too. And that makes sense. Because the remaining fiber in apples is known as insoluble fiber. This type of fiber is thought to prevent certain types of cancer. A *health bonus:* health-boosting apples are a good source of the mineral boron, which may help prevent the calcium loss from bone that may lead to brittle bone disease.

Sweet Vinegar Fact!

Apple cider vinegar, a "fruity" flavored vinegar, is often used in pickling. It's produced from fermented apple juice and is a good choice for salads and pickling. Each fall, Heinz U.S.A. purchases more than 23 million pounds of apples for vinegar production at its Holland, Michigan, factory.

POTASSIUM: THE MIRACLE WORKER OF ACV

Apple cider vinegar, again, which is made from healthful apples, contains 240 milligrams of potassium per cup. And medical experts emphasize the importance of regulating the sodium-potassium balance in our nervous and muscular systems. Potassium counteracts the damaging effects of too much sodium and can help prevent high blood pressure. This powerful mineral inhibits fluid retention, too, which is caused by an accumulation of sodium in the body. As a result, this also helps ward off high blood pressure.

Healing apple cider vinegar is also believed to help prevent energy diseases. Folk medicine doctors claim that preventable diseases or conditions such as high blood pressure, impaired memory, and even fatigue can be helped by apple cider vinegar because of its energizing potassium.

While a well-balanced diet is essential for staying power, loading up on complex carbohydrates, protein, iron, and potassium-rich foods can help you perk up *and* slim down. "Nutrient-dense foods maintain your energy levels, which helps stave off fatigue," says Jeffrey Blumberg, Ph.D., associate director of the Human Nutrition Research Center on Aging at Tufts University.

Eight Potassium-Rich Foods

Try teaming apple cider vinegar with these potassium-rich foods:

- 4 oz broiled chicken = 350–500 mg of potassium
- 1 cup dried apples = 350–500 mg of potassium
- ½ cup dried apricots = 500–750 mg of potassium
- 1 potato = 500–750 mg of potassium
- 1 cup broccoli = 350–500 mg of potassium
- 1 cup collard greens = 500–750 mg of potassium
- 1 cup low-fat yogurt with fruit = 350–500 mg of potassium
- 1 cup canned tomatoes = 500–750 mg of potassium

(Source: The Healing Foods: The Ultimate Authority of the Curative Power of Nutrition by Patricia Hausman and Judith Benn Hurley [Rodale Press, 1989].)

It's the potassium that helps energize you. Low potassium levels bring on fatigue. You need a daily minimum of 1,875 milligrams of potassium, and apple cider vinegar can help you get that.

Doctors Paul and Patricia Bragg note in their book that potassium-rich apple cider vinegar is the key to good health and longevity, too. One of the best ways to prevent age-related illnesses is by eating a healthy diet, one that is chock-full of those foods that are potassium-rich. And apple cider vinegar is one of the best—and cheapest—sources of potassium.

The Braggs describe potassium as "the mineral of youthfulness." And, they add, potassium is so important that without it there would be no life on Earth. Yet today millions of people struggle without realizing that their quality of health would be better by alleviating their potassium deficiency.[5]

I remember what it was like to watch my mother suffer. She was an alcoholic. The doctor prescribed high blood pressure medication *and* a potassium liquid to take daily. Every morning my father would fix a cranberry juice and potassium cocktail for my mom to drink. Evidently, the taste of the medicine was so bad she refused to drink it. I can't help but wonder if a well-balanced diet, less alcohol, and more exercise—plus taking potassium-rich apple cider vinegar—could have helped my mother live a longer life. She died at age 52.

Potassium helps if you are malnourished. If a disease, such as alcoholism, has progressed to where it has damaged the body's metabolism (as in the case of my mother), you would need extra potassium to keep the potassium-sodium ratio in balance for proper bodily functioning, explains Connie Diekman, R.D., an American Dietetic Association spokesperson. "The biggest reason potassium and sodium need to be in direct balance in the body is to ensure that muscles can contract and relax. The heart is the major muscle in the body, so when these two minerals are out of sync, the heart muscle can beat irregularly, which can result in heart failure."

Since Dr. Jarvis began celebrating the benefits of potassium-rich apple cider vinegar, medical experts have confirmed that it is vital for good health to maintain the proper ratio of potassium to sodium in your diet. The perfect potassium to sodium ratio is 5:1; but unfortunately most Americans have a ratio of 1:2. That means we consume twice as much sodium as we do potassium. Thanks to a modern, fast-

Do *You* Have A Potassium Deficiency?

When there is a deficiency of potassium, these symptoms can occur:
muscle weakness, fatigue, mental confusion, heart rhythm disturbances, and problems with nerve conduction. And note, potassium deficiency occurs when the body is losing more potassium than it is taking in and usually through loss in the urine, excessive perspiration, or with severe vomiting or diarrhea.

paced society, we eat more processed foods today, so our salt intake is higher, and potassium consumption is shrinking. And more Americans are growing unhealthier. Apple cider vinegar is a great way to bring back potassium, the way it used to be when we ate whole, natural foods such as vegetables and fruits, which are naturally potassium-rich.

This ratio can be imbalanced by excessive consumption of sodium, along with a low intake of potassium. An out-of-whack potassium-sodium ratio can lead to high blood pressure, heart disease, and even strokes.

Health Fact!

Attention Coffee Drinkers: Alcohol, coffee, tea, and sugar are diuretics and therefore potassium drainers. If you drink too much coffee, you might find yourself feeling fatigued. The cause: It depletes your body's required potassium.

"Only five percent of Americans' sodium intake comes from the salt shaker. Ninety-five percent of Americans' sodium intake comes from hidden sodium from the packaged foods," says Jan McBarron, M.D. Apple cider vinegar gives you more potassium so that you maintain your sodium-potassium ratio levels.

Vinegar Is Sodium-Free

While vinegar is high in potassium, it is low in sodium! After sampling a number of vinegar products, the United States Department of Agriculture reports that an average serving size, a tablespoon of vinegar, contains just a trace of sodium. That means, according to labeling guidelines for sodium in foods, vinegar is a "sodium-free" product.

Six Super Health-Promoting ACV Components

A friend of Angelo (the senior who drinks his daily apple cider vinegar cocktails), Erminia Marcini,* 60, who lives in San Jose, California, is starting to worry about age-related diseases, from arthritis to cancer. Erminia says she is eating a healthy diet—but what else can she do?

All women and men need an adequate amount of many other essential minerals and vitamins to help the body maintain good health. Experts urge people of all ages to get plenty of nutrients. Apple cider vinegar contains some of them:

1 **Beta-carotene for Healthier Cells:** Beta-carotene, a carotenoid, and trace element found in apple cider vinegar, is a potent antioxidant. This vitamin will help neutralize the free radical molecules that cause normal cells to become cancerous.

   Foods rich in beta-carotene are sweet potatoes, carrots, and spinach. Team the apple cider vinegar in our Garden Vegetable Potpourri (see page 209) with baby carrots and seasoned apple cider vinegar, and you get beta-carotene in a one-two punch.

2 **Get Your Boron:** This important trace element, which is found in apple cider vinegar, is essential for good health and strong bones. Boron plays a major role in utilizing calcium and magnesium, which are necessary for beating bone loss, too. Still, most Americans are probably not getting enough of this bone-building buddy.

You can get more boron by eating boron-rich foods such as apples. Just make up a batch of our Apple Chutney (see page 162), which is brimming with red tart apples and apple cider vinegar.

3 **Bone Up with Calcium:** Apple cider vinegar contains a trace of needed calcium. This mineral is necessary for transmitting nerve impulses and regulating muscle contraction. If your diet is deficient in calcium, the body will steal it out of your bones. This, in turn, weakens your skeleton and can lead to brittle bone disease.

"Calcium is the primary mineral in your bones. That is what keeps them strong," says Georgia Kostas, director of nutrition at the Cooper Clinic in Dallas. "It is critical to the physical structure as well as functioning of the human body."

Note these important calcium facts:

- Ninety-nine percent of the body's calcium is stored in your bones and teeth.
- One percent is in blood and tissues.
- It is necessary for transmitting nerve impulses and regulating muscle contraction.
- The need for calcium starts in infancy and continues throughout life. If your diet is deficient in calcium, the body will steal it out of your bones. This weakens your skeleton and can lead to brittle bone disease.

While apple cider vinegar may only contain a trace element of bone-building calcium, you can add it to calcium-rich dishes. Try our Pasta Primavera Salad (see page 201), which includes broccoli florets, Monterey Jack cheese, and apple cider vinegar. That way you are adding extra tangy flavor to calcium-boosting sources and keeping your bones healthy too.

4 **Enzymes for Good Digestion:** "They're protein molecules and they're what actually digest the food you eat. You can only get enzymes by eating plant foods—live food such as apples, and apple cider vinegar," explains Dr. McBarron.

What better way to get enzymes than eating plenty of fresh fruits and vegetables tossed in enzyme-rich apple cider vinegar.

May I suggest indulging in our Fast Fabulous Coleslaw. Not only is this one of my personal favorites, it's packed with live foods such as cabbage, carrots, red peppers, and apple cider vinegar.

5 **Boost Your Fiber:** When vinegar is made from fresh apples, it contains pectin or soluble fiber. Soluble fiber blocks fat absorption, which lowers blood cholesterol and reduces risk of heart disease and high blood pressure.

Naturally, foods that are fiber-plentiful will help you reach your daily fiber intake. Our Green Bean and Potato Salad will help take you there. It's full of fiber-rich beans and potatoes tossed in apple cider vinegar.

6 **Pump Up Your Iron:** Your body needs iron. Apple cider vinegar delivers iron in an easy to digest and absorbable form. Iron deficiency anemia is a common problem and can easily be avoided.

It is estimated that 240,000 toddlers and 3.3 million women suffer iron-deficiency anemia, according to researchers at the National Center for Health Statistics in Hyattsville, Maryland.

ACV's Nutrient Source Chart

While apple cider vinegar contains these nutrients, so do these nutrient-dense foods, which can be enhanced even more by using natural apple cider vinegar or herbal apple cider vinegar in our tasty recipes at the end of this book.

Beta-carotene: carrots, asparagus, broccoli, red pepper, and green leafy vegetables.

Boron: apples.

Calcium: broccoli and green leafy vegetables, tofu.

Enzymes: carrots, apples, red peppers.

Fiber: beans, potatoes.

Iron: raisins, asparagus, leafy green vegetables, spinach, kale.

Potassium: apples, onion, garlic, green leafy vegetables.

Rather than go to straight to liver, you can enjoy our Pineapple Raisin Sauce (see page 166), which contains iron-rich raisins and apple cider vinegar to help you boost your iron intake with a smile.

OTHER ACV INGREDIENTS

Not only does apple cider vinegar contain plenty of vitamins, minerals, and potassium—it contain carbohydrates and amino acids which are essential to boost brain power and other important healthful components.

Carbohydrates Supply Mental Energy. The brain needs many different kinds of nutrients—vitamins, minerals, and carbohydrates. We know that carbohydrates, which are found in apples and apple cider vinegar, are broken down by the body into the brain's most important food—glucose, a basic sugar.

Carbohydrates enhance mental performance because your brain requires glucose all of the time. It provides your brain with the energy it requires to think. A daily intake of complex carbohydrates from a host of foods (vegetables, fruits, whole grains) and apple cider vinegar are important for mental performance.

Amino Acids and Brain Chemistry. Welcome to the world of amino acids, the building blocks of all protein molecules. There are 22 amino acids—14 of these can be made by the body; thus they're considered "nonessential." The remaining 8 amino acids must be obtained from our diets; thus they're considered "essential."

Is the concept of "brain food" just wishful thinking? If an apple a day keeps the doctor away, can a cup of apple cider make us rocket scientists? Although that may sound farfetched, scientists now say that we can indeed refuel our brain power with certain nutrients that promote clearer thinking and mental energy.

The brain, like any part of the body, depends on fuel to ensure peak performance. Your brain cells communicate by releasing neurotransmitters or "smart" nutrients that relay a message to other cells in the brain and your body. Thus, essential compounds in foods contribute to the brain's own "smart" chemicals.

Studies show that when people become deficient in one or more of these nutrients, cognitive functioning becomes impaired. Correcting these deficiencies helps us feel better and function optimally. And that's where good nutrition—including apple cider vinegar, a source of brain food—comes into play.

Apple cider vinegar is believed to contain amino acids; however, it is unknown how many and which ones. Scientists are constantly finding new amino acids that the body needs to stay healthy. Although it is not put on the label, it does indeed contain trace elements of amino acids—which are essential to brain chemistry and emotion. (See Chapter 10: "Healthy Rice Vinegar.")

Alkaline/Acid Balance. In addition, natural vinegar can affect your body's pH, or acid/alkaline balance in a number of ways:

- You can change the pH of the vaginal environment at the first sign of a pesky yeast infection by turning to a natural vinegar-and-water douche. (See Chapter 15: "Therapeutic Uses.")
- In folk medicine natural healers often prescribe lemon juice and cider vinegar for detoxification and purification of the body. They have been recommended as alkalinizing agents because of their purported high content of alkaline minerals, reports Susan Lark, M.D., a preventive health doctor in Los Altos, California.[6]
- Apple cider vinegar is used to treat skin ailments such as acne and warts. Its pH (the number that indicates how much acid or alkaline is present in a solution) is identical to normal, healthy skin. It's believed that applying apple cider vinegar to skin areas will help normalize the pH on skin and speed up healing.

Hydrochloric Acid. Apple cider vinegar also helps the stomach to produce hydrochloric acid, which aids digestion. We lose acid as we age, a big reason to take apple cider vinegar to prevent digestion disorders as we get older.

"As we get older, the symptoms of lack of acid are the same as too much acid," explains Dr. Earl Mindell. For instance, indigestion may arise from either excess acid or insufficient acid in the stomach (which leads to poor digestion). "You want to have a balance. That's why a little apple cider vinegar before a meal or with a meal can help produce enough acidity that will help the normal digestion."

Dr. Jan McBarron, a dedicated diet doctor, agrees. "Vinegar is an acid—acid helps dissolve things. In order for our food to be truly digested it has to be broken down 100 percent to a pure liquid. That's the only way the small intestine can absorb the nutrients—it has to be in total liquid form," she explains. And vinegar does the trick.

I can personally attest to that. A while ago, for dinner I ordered a cobb salad. Instead of a high-fat blue cheese dressing, I opted for a red wine vinegar. The result? After my meal, rather than feeling bogged down as I have in the past with blue cheese, I felt light and energized. It was like switching from whole milk to low-fat milk. You can't go back. And I won't.

Purifying Apple Cider Vinegar. The acetic acid in apple cider vinegar is believed to help detoxify the body from foreign substances such as drugs and alcohol. And many medical doctors and folk remedy users believe vinegar—internally and externally— helps to purify your body's system.

"It unites the toxic substances with other molecules to produce a new compound. The combination of sulfanomides with acetate forms a compound that is biologically inactive and more easily excreted," reports Dr. F. Lipman of the Biochemical Research Laboratory of Massachusetts General Hospital.[7]

ACV Health Boosters

What It Is and Does	Diseases It Prevents
ACID: aids in proper digestion of food.	Digestive disorders such as heartburn and gas.
AMINO ACIDS	Impaired memory.
BETA-CAROTENE: contains carotenoids, which the liver converts into vitamin A, a cancer-fighting antioxidant.	Cancer: when your body doesn't get adequate beta-carotene, you are more likely to develop cancer of the lung, stomach, or mouth. Smokers are at a higher risk for lung and mouth cancers.
BORON: works like estrogen to prevent loss of mineral from bone; aids in utilization of vitamin D.	Osteoporosis.

CALCIUM: maintains strong, healthy bones and teeth, which store 99% of the body's calcium; helps enzymes in fat and protein digestion and energy production; helps regulate contraction of muscles, including the heart; aids absorption of other nutrients.	Osteoporosis.
ENZYMES: aid food digestion.	Digestive disorders such as poor metabolism.
FIBER	Heart disease, cancer (colon, breast).
GLUCOSE	Impaired brain power.
IRON: plays a role in immune system functioning and is important to cognition.	Anemia, fatigue.
MAGANESE: necessary for maintaining normal cholesterol levels.	Heart disorders, high cholesterol.
POTASSIUM	Fatigue, high blood pressure, heart disease, strokes, and fatigue.

It's clear that ACV has a powerhouse of health-promoting nutrients. But how exactly does this golden liquid help your body to prevent disease? Researchers and real people will show you how this nutritional wonder can help you—without ill side effects or a high cost.

Important Healing Hints to Remember

- ✓ Apple cider vinegar contains plenty of healthful nutrients.
- ✓ The quality of vinegar counts. Natural, organic, and made the slow Orleans method are recommended by folk medicine doctors.
- ✓ Apples, a component of apple cider vinegar, are fiber-rich and potassium-plentiful.
- ✓ Potassium, the miracle worker of apple cider vinegar, helps keep the body's sodium-potassium levels in balance.
- ✓ Apple cider vinegar contains beta-carotene, boron, calcium, enzymes, fiber, and iron.
- ✓ Other good stuff is in apple cider vinegar such as carbohydrates and amino acids.
- ✓ Apple cider vinegar can aid in maintaining your body's acid/alkaline balance.
- ✓ Hydrochloric acid in apple cider vinegar can help aid digestion.
- ✓ Apple cider vinegar can help your body to excrete toxins, which purifies your system.
- ✓ The total ingredients of apple cider vinegar can help prevent health ailments such as fatigue and poor digestion and ward off heart disease and cancer.

CHAPTER

5

Why Is Apple Cider Vinegar So Healthy?

A loaf of bread the Walrus said,
Is what we chiefly need:
Pepper and vinegar besides
Are very good indeed
Now if you're ready, Oysters dear,
We can begin to feed.

—Lewis Carrol[1]

Five years ago, Jan McBarron woke up at her regular time. Rather than pouring herself a cup of coffee, she had 2 tablespoons of vinegar in a glass of water. Then, while clad in leotards and a T-shirt, she ran three miles for her A.M. exercise routine.

Today, Dr. McBarron, a weight-loss specialist, uses this same energizing ritual every other day before she goes to work. It's the perfect stay-slim, keep-healthy therapy for the doctor who specializes in overweight disorders.

Do you want to be feel energized? Do you feel like your weight is out of control? Do you have skyrocketing cholesterol levels? Are you suffering from high blood pressure? If you answered "yes" to any of these questions, apple cider vinegar may be the solution to help you cope, too.

FIGHTING FAT WITH APPLE CIDER VINEGAR

"If I could do it, anyone can." That's what Dr. McBarron assures the patients who come to her with seemingly hopeless weight problems. And they believe her, because they know she's speaking from experience. Ten years ago, Dr. McBarron dropped 70 pounds from her 5 foot10 frame—and she's kept the weight off.

For a decade, Dr. McBarron fought a battle with her weight. "I lost 50 pounds—five times!" she says. "I tried every diet you can name. I'd finally attained my dream of becoming a doctor, but I was miserable because I weighed over 200 pounds! It was time to get off the roller coaster," Dr. McBarron says. And vinegar—both apple cider vinegar and red wine vinegar—is part of her meal plan that has helped her and her patients lose weight and keep it off.

Staying lean is a big health concern for Americans today. And it should be. Excess body fat is linked to killer diseases—such as high blood pressure, diabetes, stroke, and heart attack. Despite the danger of fat, losing weight is not easy. Americans are losing the battle of the bulge.

THE SKINNY ON AVC

But apple cider vinegar comes to the rescue. Doctors can vouch for this. People from coast to coast will tell you that they know about the weight loss–apple cider vinegar connection. Folks will religiously drink a tablespoon of apple cider vinegar, especially raw (unpasturized) and organic in a glass of warm water every morning because they believe it will help them to lose pounds, boost energy, and aid digestion.

Meanwhile, I have not heard of any groundbreaking, controlled weight-loss studies in this country that document apple cider vinegar as a weight-loss aid. However, research does show how apple cider vinegar's fat-fighting ingredients—such as fiber—can indeed help pare excess pounds.

Furthermore, the fiber and nutrients in apple cider vinegar can help keep you healthy if you are watching your caloric intake. Both apples and apple cider vinegar contain pectin, a type of fiber found mostly in fruits. It can help suppress a runaway appetite.

Here's proof: Scientists at the University of Southern California found that adding 15 grams of concentrated pectin to the meals of nine overweight people delayed the time required for food to leave their stomachs by 45 minutes. The reason: Pectin plumps up food as it's processed by the stomach, boosting feelings of fullness and suppressing the appetite. The pectin-rich meals helped the people in the study to eat less and shed more than 6½ pounds in one month.[2]

And some people, who mix 1 tablespoon of vinegar in a glass of water and drink the solution a half hour before meals, vow that it curbs the appetite. Could it be possible that the fiber in apple cider vinegar, like apples, fills you up?

Another boon to apple cider vinegar's slimming power is how it can keep the body's sodium-potassium levels in check. According to Dr. McBarron, when the ratio of sodium-potassium is balanced, you'll eat less, because you're not going to be as hungry.

Potassium-rich foods can help decrease unwanted water retention—and flatten the tummy, too. "Potassium works on the body to counterbalance sodium. And sodium is another factor that may cause you to retain water and feel bloated," says Terri Brownlee, R.D., M.P.H., in Durham, North Carolina. ACV and potassium-rich foods like watermelon, bananas, cantaloupe, dried apricots, and vegetables can act as natural diuretics, which may reduce bloating.

Not only is apple cider vinegar rich in pectin and potassium, it's got another fat fighter that you should know about. Acetic acid, the primary ingredient in vinegar, has long been believed to boost metabolism and to dissolve fats.

Bloat-Busting Meal Plan

This slimming, healthy meal plan—designed by New Jersey–based nutritionist Toni Gerbino—can flatten your tummy fast! Give it a try for two days before a special occasion. I tried it, and even though I am a slim 120 pounds at 5-5, it worked wonders. My tummy was flatter and I felt energized!

Breakfast: Fresh berries (no limit).

Lunch: 4 ounces fresh white meat turkey
greens with dressing made of fresh parsley, 1 tablespoon each virgin olive oil and apple cider vinegar, and spices to taste
1 cup fresh berries

Dinner: 6–8 ounces fresh flounder, sole, or salmon
asparagus with lemon, apple cider vinegar, and parsley
1 cup fresh berries

- Drink a minimum of six 8-ounce glasses of water with fresh lemon throughout the day.
- Check with your doctor before starting this or any diet.

Switch to Apple Cider Vinegar

In addition to vinegar cocktails, easy menu changes can help to melt pounds away as easy as 1-2-3. Here, take a look:

1 Switch to fat-free vinegar salad dressing. One of the biggest sources of fat and calories in the average woman's diet is salad dressing. "The main ingredient in regular salad dressing is vegetable oil, which gets 100 percent of its calories from fat," says Neva Cochran, R.D., in Dallas, Texas. When you toss a salad of mixed greens, substitute 2 tablespoons fat-free vinegar dressing for the 2 tablespoons of regular dressing you normally use three times a week.

2 You'll whittle your waistline faster when you trim your sandwich, even just a little. Once a week, build a more slimming sandwich just by leaving out one slice of meat and the cheese, and replacing mayonnaise with vinegar. Then add flavorful, filling layers of fiber- and water-rich dark, leafy greens and tomatoes.

3 Eliminate 1 teaspoon of butter or margarine a day. Giving up just 1 teaspoon of butter or margarine a day will make a big difference. Instead of sautéing your vegetables in butter, try nonstick cooking spray and a splash of vinegar to avoid adding extra calories from fat.

ACV Fat-Fighters' Corner

Tangy apple cider vinegar is delicious. But with its other fat-fighting qualities, it is not just for salads. It's a refreshing and tasty addition to sandwiches, main dishes, and more.

- It has only 15 calories per tablespoon.
- It has no fat.
- It has no sodium.
- It's potassium-rich, which can help fight water retention.

For now, the final word on apple cider vinegar is that it can put you on the track to good health and long-term weight loss. If you really want to shed excess pounds—and enjoy long-lasting results—start eating a good, well-balanced diet, include apple cider vinegar whenever you can, and have your doctor recommend an exercise regimen suited to your goals.

Apple Cider Vinegar Helps Keep Blood Pressure in Check

As a health writer always on deadline and prone to stress-induced high blood pressure, I've taken an alternative route to staying heart-healthy. Each day I make sure I get plenty of fruits and vegetables—and now, vinegar is also part of my prescription to good health.

As people age, they become more susceptible to several life-threatening diseases. According to the American Heart Association, about one out of four adults has high blood pressure. Untreated high blood pressure can bring on a deadly stroke or heart attack.

Rather than opt for medication, apple cider vinegar can aid in the prevention of high blood pressure, and today, doctors know that potassium—which we already know ACV is rich in—is needed to counteract the damaging effects of sodium—including high blood pressure.

Health Fact!

If your blood pressure is under 140/90, there is little need for you to be overly concerned about a moderate salt intake.

The American Medical Association found that potassium lowers blood pressure. The results of 33 studies showed that potassium lowers blood pressure in patients with hypertension, and it can also help prevent hypertension by lowering blood pressure levels. While all the research was based on potassium supplements, the lead author, Dr. Paul Welton, a professor and dean of the Tulane University School of Public Health in New Orleans, believes that this is not the only way to obtain the desired level. Many fruits and vegetables are potassium-rich, and eating five or six a day can fill the recommended intake of potassium.

Good Potassium-Rich Fruits for Keeping Your Blood Pressure Lower

Vinegars can be made from the various fruits below. (See Part 4, "Other Natural Vinegars.")

1 apple = 159 mg	1 orange = 237 mg
3 apricots = 313 mg	1 peach = 171 mg
1 cup blueberries = 129 mg	1 pear = 208 mg
1 cup cranberries = 67 mg	1 plum = 113 mg
1 lemon = 80 mg	1 pomegranate = 399 mg
1 mango = 322 mg	1 cup raspberries = 187 mg
	1 cup strawberries = 247 mg

Avoid These High Blood Pressure Culprits

Bacon	Marinated foods*	Smoked food	High-sodium canned foods
Catsup	Diet soda	Fast food	Ham
Hot dogs	Pickled foods*	Salted potato chips	Salted pretzels
Salted nuts	Fried food	Sausage	Shellfish
Fatty meats	Seasoned salts	Duck, goose	Butter

*If your blood pressure is normal, go ahead and enjoy seasoned salts, and eat marinated and/or pickled foods in moderation.

The Vinegar and Fiber–Cholesterol Connection

Heart problems are a major problem to both men and women. Apple cider vinegar can be heart-healthy too, because it contains pectin, a soluble fiber, which aids in lowering cholesterol.

Fiber-rich apple cider vinegar can contain a healthy dose of pectin when its made from fresh, natural apples. "Soluble fiber helps reduce cholesterol by binding it with the fiber, which your body then eliminates," says Connie Diekman, R.D. This, in turn, reduces the risk of heart ailments, such as heart attacks and strokes.

The Cholesterol Puzzle

Dazed and confused about cholesterol? Here's the lowdown. The more high-density lipoproteins or HDL (good cholesterol) you have, the better. This kind we want to be high—it lowers the risk of heart disease. Oxidized (free radical–damaged), LDL (bad cholesterol) puts you at higher risk for heart disease. But you can guard against it with antioxidant vitamins which are found in apple cider vinegar.

Anticancer Apple Cider Vinegar

Cancer: It is a frightening disease for men, women, children, and pets. And today it is the second most deadly disease. So what exactly is cancer? It is a group of diseases characterized by abnormal cells that go awry. If the spread is not controlled, you can die.

Cancer is caused by external (chemicals, radiation, and viruses) and internal (hormones, immune conditions, and inherited mutations) factors, according to the American Cancer Society. But you can reduce the risk of getting cancer.

Scientists now know that dietary changes hold the key to preventing a number of cancers, and research shows that certain antioxidant-rich fruits and vegetables—especially teamed with apple cider vinegar, which contains beta-carotene, a carotenoid—can help guard against cancers.

"Moreover, carotenoids serve as the body's raw material for the production of vitamin A, another potent antioxidant, the scarcity of which has been linked, in particular, to cancers of the respiratory system, colon and bladder. Carotenoids and vitamin A work in concert to protect the body from cancers associated with chemical toxins," explains Dr. Earl Mindell.[3]

Numerous studies have found that eating fruits and vegetables cuts the risk of cancer. Medical experts know that eating foods high in the antioxdants C, E, and beta-carotene may trap free radical molecules that cause normal cells to become cancerous.

The National Cancer Institute recommends you get between 20 and 30 grams of fiber a day by eating a diet high in fruits, vegetables, and whole grains. Pectin, a soluble fiber in vinegar, helps dilute cancer-causing compounds in your body and speed cancer-causing dietary fats through the colon before they can be absorbed, according to research. In fact, studies show that a high fiber diet can kill colon cells, report British Medical researchers in London.[4]

But no single food or supplement can prevent cancer. Apple cider vinegar, which contains both beta carotene and fiber, is not a magic bullet—it's still very important to eat a variety of antioxidant-rich fruits and vegetables to reduce all cancers.

Cancer is the disease that is most feared by mature adults. Breast cancer and prostate cancer are among the seven deadliest cancers. And they both are very sensitive medical matters.

The bad news is breast cancer is second only to lung cancer in cancer deaths. By age 85 one in nine women will contract breast cancer. And prostate cancer is the leading cancer among American men. All men are at risk for developing prostate cancer. The average age of diagnosis is 65, according to the National Cancer Institute.

But the good news is both hormonally driven cancers are preventable—and almost always curable when caught early.

• **Breast Cancer:** Risk of breast cancer, reported the American Cancer Society (ACS), is linked to various factors that affect circulating hormone levels throughout life: age of menstruation, number of pregnancies, breastfeeding, obesity, and physical activity. Here's the best dietary approach to risk reduction:

A low-fat diet (one with 30 percent or less of total calories coming from fat) may keep "bad" estrogen (a female hormone) levels down, limiting exposure to the type of estrogen that leads tumor growth.

Instead of high-fat toppings and high-fat food, pile your plate with fruits and vegetables and use vinegar when it's palatable. Remember the label on ACV? It shows that this product can help you to lower your caloric intake and maintain a low-fat diet.

As an alternative to high-fat meat, try soy foods. Genistein, a compound in soybeans, may be able to inhibit the spreading of cancerous tumors. It is believed that it inhibits the growth of new blood vessels which nourish cancer cells. So start snacking on more soy nuts, soy milk, soy burgers, and miso soup. (See Honey Miso Sauce, page 193.)

Eating more vegetables. For added protection, follow the NCI guidelines to eat five or more servings of fruits and vegetables—especially vegetables from the cabbage family, such as broccoli, cauliflower, and Brussels sprouts. In fact, studies show that cruciferous veggies have a chemical called indole-3-carbinol which helps to decrease the levels of the "bad" estrogen like a low-fat diet does. And note, teaming fruits and vegetables with beta-carotene-rich apple cider vinegar may prevent cancer, too.

• **Prostate Cancer:** Scientists know that prostate cancer is connected to male hormones, but they are unclear as to the exact mechanism which causes the cancer. Here's the best dietary approach to risk reduction.

The best preventive measure, according to the American Cancer Society, is to limit intake of foods from animal sources, especially saturated fats and red meats. Lean poultry such as turkey and chicken with whole grains such as brown rice and pasta are good substitutes. And note, our meal plans boast slim and healthy eating with flavorful apple cider vinegar.

Switching to low-fat fare based on fresh vegetables and fruit which are chock-full of the antioxidant vitamins C, E, and beta-carotene (again, which is present in apple cider vinegar) will help protect against prostate cancer by trapping cancer-causing free radical molecules.

• **Cervical Cancer:** The rates of cervical cancer have plummeted over the past decades, according to the American Cancer Society. The lower rates are due to the Papanicolaou (Pap) test, which was introduced in the 1950s.

Recently researchers at Johns Hopkins University in Baltimore and the University of Zimbabwe found vinegar could screen for cervical cancer where Pap tests aren't available. The low-cost technique could improve the chances of detecting cancer in developing countries such as Asia, Latin America, and Africa.

Nurse-midwives used the vinegar technique to screen 10,934 women at primary-care clinics in Zimbabwe. Precancerous cells turn white when swabbed with an applicator soaked in a solution of acetic acid, the main ingredient in vinegar. Pap smears were also performed on the women and the vinegar test was more likely to pick up precancerous or cancercous cells than the pap smear.[5]

While cervical cancer in the United States has decreased, about 4,800 women are expected to die of it each year. The study's coauthor Paul Blumenthal often sees patients with an abnormal Pap smear. He may repeat the Pap smear, but he will also splash vinegar on the cervix as a backup test. To me this is good news. As a DES daughter (DES, a synthetic estrogen given to about 4.8 million women in the United States between 1938 and 1971, has been linked to a rare form of cancer in their daughters), I know what abnormal Pap smears are all about. Who would have thought vinegar could be used as a "second opinion"?

In conclusion, according to the American Institute for Cancer Research, scientists have not yet pinpointed how dietary fat promotes cancer development. However, it seems that fat is involved in both the early abnormal cell changes that may lead to cancer and in helping existing tumors to grow. For now, research shows that dietary changes are your best safeguard against cancer.

ACV Cancer-Prevention Nutrients

While apple cider vinegar contains beta-carotene, vitamin C, and calcium, it can also be paired with these cancer-fighting nutrients found in foods in our recipes:

Nutrient	Found in	What It Does	Protection
Beta-carotene	Carrots, salad greens	Beta-carotene in the body can change into retinoic acid, a substance used	Stomach, larynx, lung, esophagus,

		to treat cancer of the blood and bladder	breast
Vitamin C	Broccoli, strawberries, red and green peppers	Boosts protective white cell activity	Breast, stomach
Calcium	Tofu	Calcium, in association with vitamin D, binds to fats in the intestine, reducing ability to promote cancer	Colon

Scientists' Anticancer Marinade

So you probably know that meats cooked at high temperatures on a grill form cancer-causing compounds, right? Well, I bet you don't know that a recipe from researchers at Lawrence Livermore National Laboratory in California offers a solution. While studying the effects of chemicals in our diet, they found a new way to lower "bad" compounds called heterocyclic amines.

"When we barbecued market-fresh meat, we found startlingly high levels of heterocyclic amines," says Jim Felton, Ph.D., division leader in molecular and structural biology. But when Felton and his colleagues coated chicken with a special marinade before grilling it, the results changed. They still don't know exactly how it decreases the heterocylcic amines—but it works.

Here's the scientists anticancer marinade: ½ cup packed brown sugar, 3 cloves crushed garlic, 1½ teaspoons salt, 3 tablespoons mustard, ¼ cup cider vinegar, 3 tablespoons lemon juice, and 6 tablespoons olive oil.

Apple Cider Vinegar Beats Bone Loss

The statistics are frightening. One in two women and one in eight men over age 50 will have an osteoporosis-related fracture in their lifetime. But as scary as this seems, we are not powerless. The right nutrient-dense diet—teamed with apple cider vinegar, which contains bone builders such as boron and calcium—can help lower our risk.

According to Vikki Petersen, D.C., in San Jose, California, evidence shows that boron, a bone-buddy mineral, plays a role in utilizing calcium and magnesium—other bone builders. Still, most Americans are probably not getting enough boron, which is found in apple cider vinegar.

"Boron deficiency may be associated with an increased risk for post-menopausal bone loss. Boron deprivation in post-menopausal women leads to increased urinary excretion of calcium and magnesium," adds Petersen.

Boron also helps the metabolism of calcium and magnesium—and boosts blood levels of the bone-building hormones estrogen and testosterone, according to research by Dr. Forest Nielsen of the U.S. Department of Agriculture Research Service in Grand Forks, North Dakota.

The RDA is not set, but recent U.S. research suggests 2 to 3 mg. Your best bets: soy, prunes, and apples.

In addition, most women don't get the recommended daily allowance of bone-building calcium in their diet. Experts say the average American woman takes in about 400 to 500 mg per day. Yet an adult woman 25 to 50 years of age needs 1000 mg.

But apple cider vinegar comes to the rescue again. If taking a tablespoon of vinegar in water doesn't appeal to you, try more calcium-rich recipes that include broccoli, or tofu such as in our bone-boosting Tofu and Toasted Peanut Salad (see page 187) paired with apple cider vinegar.

Boosting Your Memory with Apple Cider Vinegar

Iron, a mineral found in apple cider vinegar, may strengthen brain power. Since iron is involved in distributing oxygen to brain cells (and every other cell in the body), when you lack this mineral you find it hard to concentrate.

IMPORTANT HEALING HINTS TO REMEMBER

ACV KEEPS THE DOCTOR AWAY

Disease	How ACV Works
✓ Overweight	Fiber in ACV provides bulk/curbs appetite; keeps sodium-potassium ratio in balance so you're less hungry and decreases bloating and water retention.
✓ High blood pressure	Potassium in ACV helps reduce high blood pressure.
✓ High cholesterol	Insoluble fiber in ACV reduces cholesterol by binding with fiber, which is eliminated by body.
✓ Cancer	Beta-carotene in ACV helps fight cancer-causing free radicals in the body and boosts the immune system; acetic acid in vinegar helps detect cervical cancer.
✓ Osteoporosis	Boron in ACV helps metabolize bone-builders calcium and magnesium; calcium helps keeps bones strong.
✓ Impaired memory	Iron and boron in ACV are needed to keep mental functioning at its best.

In the early 1990s, Harold Sandstead, M.D., professor of preventive medicine at the University of Texas, discovered that women whose diets lack zinc and iron experienced more difficulties on standard exams than women with an adequate dietary supply. In his study of women aged 18 to 40, Sandstead found that giving these women more zinc and iron raised their scores on memory tests and average of 20 percent.

Boron plays a crucial part in memory function, too. Scientists at the USDA's Human Nutrition Research Center have linked boron deficiencies to chronic lethargy and fatigue. In brain studies, they found that the electrical activity of the gray matter in the boron-deficient indicated increased drowsiness and mental sluggishness.

Food for thought? Your best food sources for these two nutrients to help strengthen your mental powers: Boron: apples, broccoli, cabbage, cauliflower. Iron: ground beef, turkey, spinach, and peas. To get you started, try our apple cider vinegar recipes: Fast Fabulous Coleslaw and Sweet and Sour Meat Balls.

PART 3

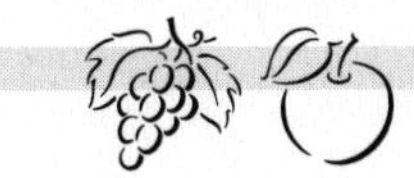

Red Wine Vinegar

CHAPTER

6

The Red Wine Vinegar Chronicle

Beware of vinegar of sweete wine, and the anger of a peaceable man.

—John Florio, First Fruits[1]

While apple cider vinegar may hold forefront in U.S. history, wine vinegar, its ignored counterpart, was commonly used as well in the past centuries. Wine vinegar, naturally, is made from wine—red, white, or rosé—and is medicinal from head to toe as well.

In 5,000 B.C., the Babylonians used grapes to make vinegar. Hippocrates, tagged "the father of medicine," used wine vinegar as an antibiotic to treat his patients in 400 B.C. The Four Thieves used vinegar during the plague in Marseilles. Throughout time, wine vinegar, like apple cider vinegar, was a cure-all folk remedy.

Generations of families, rich and poor, have used wine vinegar to help remedy a wide range of ailments—both inside and outside the body. Red wine vinegar, a sacred and mysterious cure-all for thousands of years, has been a medicine, a preservative, and a primary cooking ingredient to the folks of the Mediterranean.

At the opposite corner of Castile (due south of the Basque country) in Rioja is the region of Spain's best red wine vineyards. This is one of the original places where red wine vinegar is made. Yet while folk medicine has been busy touting apple cider vinegar throughout American history, it has ignored the vast virtues of its forerunner—red wine vinegar, an ancient medicinal miracle, too.

A New Look at an Old Vinegar

Red wine vinegar was used centuries ago for its antiseptic and antibacterial healing qualities. Recently, I eagerly spoke to vinegar aficionado Lawrence Diggs, author of *Vinegar*, who chatted up some new ideas on old wine vinegars.

Which doctors, besides Hippocrates, turned to red wine vinegar for its healing power? "Who knows," he says. "If you have a fine red wine vinegar, you're probably not going to be using it to clean out your stomach." However, he adds, doctors might resort to wine vinegar for treatment if that's all they had on hand. "But they would probably use vinegar from a cheaper thing. Because all you need is an acetic acid. That's what's working in terms of antiseptic."

According to Diggs, Hippocrates did not use apple cider vinegar. "It was wine vinegar." The odds are good that the good doctor used wine vinegar as an antibiotic to treat his patients, he says. "One would guess it was wine vinegar because the Greeks and Romans were into wine."

For example, it has been reported that vinegar was part of the reason that the Roman army succeeded. It is believed that Spartianus, a Latin historian, documented that vinegar mixed with water was the drink that helped the soldiers survive battle as well as the various climates they endured in Europe, Asia, and Africa. Undiluted vinegar was easier to transport than wine, and also more sobering.

Red wine vinegar also should be given credit for the Middle Ages. Remember the four robbers who were able to rob from the dead and dying without getting sick by dousing themselves with Four Thieves Vinegar? Well, apple cider vinegar may not have been the key lifesaving ingredient, after all.

"I think it was wine vinegar because that was the common vinegar in that time and place—in most of Europe. The place people talk about The Plague is France and Italy, and those places have a lot of wine," says Diggs. "We know that the vinegar that was most common at that time was wine vinegar. Now whether it was *red wine vinegar*, we don't know."

Vinegar for Self-Preservation

In 1803 Ivan Gyodorovich Kruzenshlern, a Russia navigator and explorer, set out on an exploration of the globe. To prevent scurvy, he had a large amount of vitamin C–rich cabbage pickled in barrels and brought them onboard his ship before he left for sea.

In 1806 he and most of his crewmen were in good health. The secret? Vegetable oil and cabbage soaked in vinegar. There was no record of what kind of vinegar he used to make pickled cabbage. It was believed, however, that he used natural wine vinegar since there was no synthetic vinegar made of petroleum alcohol at that time.[2]

Red Wine Vinegar: Then and Now

I remember as a young girl growing up in the fifties that red wine vinegar and oil were mainstays on our kitchen table. My mom was a wonderful cook who made meals from scratch. She saw to it that our family ate a salad with oil and red wine vinegar every day. And there's more.

When I was nine years old, my mother went to Europe for three weeks. She went to France, Italy, and Rome. When she returned, the gourmet cook inside her came out of the closet. Our family was served a vast variety of dishes from the Mediterranean world. From snails to fettuccini, wine vinegars became a permanent fixture on our table.

And today, the foods that sustain the Mediterranean table—bread, olive oil, red wine—and of course, red wine vinegar—have become mainstays of American restaurant tables and are even making it into the homes of American families—not just mine.

I can personally attest to this. Not only have I noticed small Italian restaurants boasting all-white or red-and-white-checkered tablecloths, but on each table, big or small, sure enough, there's a glass container of olive oil and red wine vinegar. And now, at home on a glass kitchen table I have the same. It adds a worldly European flair, and naturally, it's for health's sake.

While we know that apple cider vinegar is the most loved vinegar for eating, red wine vinegar is the most popular of the specialty vinegars, according to Heinz U.S.A. And doctors in America are using red wine vinegar, too, for extra flavor—*and* for health's sake.

Allan Magaziner, M.D., for one, is aware of the possibility that red wine vinegar may contain resveratrol—like wine. And since he doesn't drink, he gets the potential health perks of red wine vinegar without the ill effects of alcohol. He believes that red wine vinegar, like apple cider vinegar, contains healthful ingredients—and perhaps even more that scientists will discover in the future.

Important Healing Hints to Remember

- ✔ Wine vinegar was used as an antibiotic as early as 5,000 B.C.
- ✔ Wine vinegar was used in the Middle Ages in Europe to fight the plague.
- ✔ Red wine vinegar was derived from Spain's best red wine vineyards.
- ✔ Wine vinegar preserved food and lives back in the early 19th century.
- ✔ Today doctors use red wine vinegar regularly for its healthful antioxidant compounds.

CHAPTER

7

The Old and New Healthful Ingredients

You drink vinegar when you have wine at your elbow.

—Thomas Fuller[1]

The best red wine vinegars are believed to be made by the slow, or Orleans, process. Some vinegar companies make chemical- and additive-free red wine vinegars. They come from wines that are grown with all-natural fertilizers and without chemical pesticides, and contain no sulfites, a common food additive.

The best part is that these red wine vinegars may retain healthful nutrients. While the best red wine vinegars contain no unhealthy ingredients, they have many recognized ingredients and even "hidden" ones you should know about.

Red Wine Vinegar Nutrition Facts

If you take a look at a nutritional label of natural, organic red wine vinegar, such as Spectrum Naturals Organic Red Wine Vinegar, you will be pleasantly surprised. It will tell you that it comes from fine Italian red wines to provide a full-bodied vinegar with exceptional flavor. It reads that it's slowly aged without added sulfites. Also, it does not contain added sugar or artificial colorings. Plus, it is organically grown and processed in accordance with the California Organic Foods Act of 1990.

Per serving size—1 tablespoon—a common brand of red wine vinegar label will tell you that it contains no calories, no fat, 5 milligrams of sodium, no carbohydrates, and no protein. It is not a significant source of cholesterol, dietary fiber, vitamin A, vitamin C, calcium, or iron.

Keep in mind, however, if you analyze 3½ ounces, almost one-half cup of red wine vinegar, there will be other ingredients, based on a product data sheet by a national vinegar company: [2]

- Water: 89 grams
- Calcium: 8 grams
- Phosphorous: 10 milligrams
- Sodium: 6 milligrams
- Potassium: 80 milligrams

A New Class of Nutrients

So are you now wondering where's the good grape–red wine stuff in red wine vinegar? No one knows for sure. "It's possible that there could be some antioxidants in red wine vinegar," says UC Davis wine chemist Andrew Waterhouse, Ph.D.

"What we're looking at is a new class of antioxidants which don't have, according to governmental nutritionists, any nutritional value. And what we're trying to do, is establish whether or not they have some nutritional or health benefit," says Dr. Waterhouse.

"There's also some dispute among the people studying this whether these things could ever be called nutrients because of the definition of nutrient," adds Dr. Waterhouse. And up to now, no one has ever included these nutrients in Western medicine.

In addition, some of these new disease-fighting nutrients on the block may or may not go astray during the vinegar-making process. Because vinegar is made with a lot of oxygen and air exposure, a lot of the antioxidants found in wine are broken down, explains Dr. Waterhouse. "But I don't know how much."

He does theorize, however, that red wine vinegar, like red wine, does contain some good stuff. "The phenols that are in the grapes are probably the best for you." And past research shows exactly that.

The Grape Stuff

Wine vinegar has grapes as its raw material. Keep in mind that red wine vinegar comes from red grapes. And grapes, whether fresh, juiced, or fermented, are an excellent source of flavonoids—phenolic compounds that act as powerful antioxidants.

Flavonoids: powerful disease fighters, may help to fight viruses, allergies, carcinogens, and inflammation. In addition, these super antioxidants may also help to reduce your cholesterol level and prevent the oxidation of LDL cholesterol.

Proanthocyanidin: a flavonoid abundant in grapes.

Quercetin: a flavonoid that appears in red wine grapes, for instance, may be one of the most powerful anticancer agents ever found. It may reverse tumor growth by blocking the conversion of normal body cells to cancer cells; improves pancreas function, and levels the release of insulin; it may help prevent some problems linked with diabetes (cataracts, blindness, nerve damage, and kidney damage).

Resveratrol: another natural compound in grapes that may play a role in producing healthy cholesterol levels, reduces unhealthy fats in the blood, and prevents blood clotting in arteries narrowed by years of eating a high-fat diet.

In two European studies on the phenolic composition of high-quality wine vinegars (including "El Condado" wine vinegars and sherry vinegar) produced in the south of Spain, researchers found a variety of phenolic compounds—and a few compounds not identified in other traditional wine vinegars. However, much more research must be done.[3]

Meanwhile, "People are trying to associate red wine vinegar with red wine. They figure that the stuff is in the red wine so the logical extension is that it must be in red wine vinegar. And they're right," says Lawrence Diggs.

"The question is," he adds, "does it change when it reacts with acetic acid. Does it have the same benefits? If you put acetic acid on a sore, it will kill a lot of bacteria. However, if you drink it, the body neutralizes the acetic acid as it's on its way down. So is it as good as red wine? Who knows? We don't have the studies."

Fact: Red Wine Polyphenols Are Good for You

We know red wine is chock-full of polyphenols—those powerful antioxidants that guard against heart disease. How? Polyphenols block the oxidation of LDL or the "bad" cholesterol. Studies show that red wine polyphenols can slow down blood clotting. That means it can help lower the odds of blood clots forming which are the culprits of heart attack and stroke.

Research at the University of California at Davis also shows that red wine polyphenols slowed the formation of tumors in mice bred to develop the types of cancers that strike humans.

Also, scientists at U.C. Berkeley have shown that red wine is rich in the new class of polyphenols, powerful antioxidants that help neutralize free radicals which damage DNA, alter body chemistry, and destroy cells.

RESVERATROL

Resveratrol (pronounced *res-VER-a-trawl*), is found in both red grapes and red wine. It's another flavonoid that covers the skins of grapes and fights disease. It's also a natural fungicide that helps protect grapes from bacteria.

Grapes are one of the richest sources. "Grapes and anything made from grapes that include the grape skin or some effective extraction of the grape skin contains resveratrol. The usual example is that the resveratrol is low in white wine, not because all white grapes are low, but because the skins are discarded when white wine is made. The amount in grapes, juice and wine is different in years, locations and varieties," explains Dr. Leroy Creasy, Ph.D., emeritus professor of fruit and vegetable science at Cornell University College of Agriculture in New York.

New research indicates that resveratrol may be the ingredient in red wine which helps lower cholesterol. Resveratrol also seems to prevent blood platelet aggregation, and reduced blood clotting in arteries narrowed by years of eating a high-fat diet.

Resveratrol may also be a powerful cancer inhibitor. It may cause precancerous cells to return to normal, according to a 1997 University of Illinois study. John Pezzuto at the University of Illinois at Chicago screened about 1,000 plants for anticancer activity. He discovered one active ingredient—resveratrol. In lab tests, resveratrol zapped both cancer-inducing free radicals and inflammation.[4]

When I first spoke with Dr. Creasy, he believed that there was a good chance that red wine vinegar would indeed contain resveratrol. "Red wine vinegar made strictly from wine would probably have as much as the wine. Unless it's broken down by the bacteria and we don't know that yet." And so I waited . . .

THE TEST RESULTS

"I analyzed a cheap red wine vinegar," reports Dr. Creasy. "There was no resveratrol. The red wine vinegar profile looked like diluted red wine. Apparently diluted 10 times. It is quite likely that red wine vinegar from different producers will be distinct in phenolic composition."

The good news is, Dr. Creasy said that analyzing one red wine vinegar sample doesn't mean that much. "Because if you had pure red wine vinegar it could be there. That's based on my experience with the wine people. There isn't anything that could be absolutely certified as being 100 percent vinegar."

He added, "It is still possible that the Acetobacter organism can break down resveratrol. Resveratrol does inhibit some bacteria and possibly some have developed the biochemistry to destroy it. So it may have been there at the start but might be gone. No one knows." Currently, whether or not red wine vinegar contains resveratrol remains a very controversial topic and has not yet been scientifically proven.

Other Antioxidants and Red Wine Vinegar

Dr. Waterhouse does not know for certain if red wine vinegar does contain resveratrol. But he does know that there are a lot of polyphenols in red wine vinegar, as in red wine. "Some of the polyphenols have a good research history, other ones are called antioxidants—but they don't have any medical effect whatsoever. Antioxidants are important for health, but which specific ones are still under investigation," he says.

U.C. Davis research involves the wine compounds—tannins, quercetin, and resveratrol—found in red wines. Their studies showed that tannin-rich wine was able to reduce platelet aggregation and increase HDL cholesterol levels, suggesting that tannins may help protect against heart disease.

Can red wine vinegar do what red wine does—and more? "Certainly. In test-tube studies," answers Dr. Creasy. "Quercetin, tannins in red wine occur in all plants, including grapes, wine and probably vinegar."

In fact, for people like Dr. Creasy who don't drink alcohol, he believes including red wine vinegar in the diet would be good. "It adds up," he says. "You're supposed to eat five fruits or vegetables a day and I heard that 95 percent of Americans don't get that per day. Most people can't eat a lot of vinegar, but if you put it on veggies and your five a day you're on the healthy track."

Red wine vinegar is also the vinegar of choice for Connie Diekman, R.D. "I do use that as a seasoning on chicken, fish, salads, and marinades." Does she use it for health reasons? "I do it more as a flavoring. Because that is what we *know* it can do. And that gives pleasure to eating," she says. "But it does come from the grape and I am picking up some of the potential antioxidants."

Important Healing Hints to Remember

- ✓ The best red wine vinegars are made by the slow Orleans process.
- ✓ Red wine vinegar is no-cal, fat-free, and low in sodium.
- ✓ Red wine vinegar may contain disease-fighting antioxidants and maybe resveratrol.
- ✓ By teaming red wine vinegar with vegetables, you will get more antioxidants in your total diet.

RED WINE VINEGAR'S POTENTIAL DISEASE-FIGHTING INGREDIENTS

Ingredient	What It Does	May Help Prevent
Catechin	Blocks LDL (bad) cholesterol from entering the artery walls, inhibits blood clots, relaxes blood vessels, inhibits tumors.	High cholesterol, stroke, cancer
Polyphenols	Slow down blood clotting by its antioxidant action; inhibit formation of cancer-causing carcinogens.	Heart attack, stroke
Proanthocyanidins (PCOs)	Block the formation of cholesterol deposits on artery walls.	Heart disease
Quercetin	Reverses tumor growth by blocking the conversion of normal body cells and cancer cells; improves pancreas function, and levels the release of insulin; free radical scavenger.	Cancer; diabetes complications (e.g. cataracts and kidney damage)
Resveratrol	Prevents blood platelet aggregation and reduces blood clotting in arteries; lowers cholesterol.	Heart attack; stroke
Tannins	Reduce platelet aggregation and increase HDL cholesterol levels.	Heart disease

CHAPTER

8

Tapping Into the French Paradox

The French are not sloppy about their eating habits. They have discipline in their diet, and include plenty of fresh fruits and vegetables.

—Elisabeth Helsing, Ph.D.,
World Health Organization in Europe[1]

Did you know that heart attacks, strokes, and cancer are the three deadly diseases that account for the majority of diseases in the United States? That is why it is important for you to understand the term "French paradox"—especially when it may be one of the red wine vinegar wonders.

Medical researchers thought that reducing the fat intake and boosting the carbohydrate intake in your diet would lower your risk of heart attack and strokes. Yet the number of fat-loving diseases soars. Scientists concluded that people just consumed too much of the typical American high-fat fare. However, in France, even though the typical French citizen eats a diet richer in fat—much of it artery-clogging saturated animal fat—there is a significantly lower rate of heart disease in that country than in America where it is the Number 1 killer. This apparent inconsistency was called "The French Paradox" back in 1991 by Serge Renuade, M.D., Director of the French National Institute of Health and Medical Research.[2]

It's no secret that the French enjoy their rich sauces and fat-laden cheese. Renaude believed that part of this so-called French paradox was linked to their consumption of red wine.

Keep in mind, however, the French diet also includes a lot of antioxidant-rich garlic, fruits, and vegetables. Mealtime in France is a time for relaxing—and the French do not overeat the way men, women, and children do in America. Food portions are smaller, and the French don't eat as many Big Macs and fried chicken as Americans do.

There's More to the French Diet

According to medical experts, the French paradox is more likely due to a variety of reasons. The French eat plenty of fresh fruits and vegetables (see Chapter 13, "Combining Vinegars and Garlic, Onions, and Olive Oil"); eat in a relaxed, family-style environment; and exercise.

Researchers have now discovered that the red wine savored by the French people contains healthful chemicals such as tannins, quercetin, oligo, proanthocyanidin, catechins, and epicatechins. However, it's resveratrol that may be able to prevent the inflammation of the blood vessels and blood platelets from clumping.

But the question remains, does red wine vinegar have the same potential health effects as red wine? "Because it is derived from red wine it probably is still going to have some of the benefits as red wine, perhaps not as strong," says Dr. Allan Magaziner, one of the leading authorities in nutritional and preventative medicine. "I know red wine is studied more at this time. In the years to come, perhaps we'll find much more beneficial effects of red wine vinegar."

Red Wine versus Red Wine Vinegar

Okay, so red wine has some good health benefits. Let's look at the benefits of drinking red wine: According to Robert Crayhon, M.S., certified nutritionist, copper-containing substances are sprayed on French vineyards. Copper is a heart-healthy nutrient which helps keep cholesterol levels in normal ranges. Red wine contains powerful antioxidants. It can help relax you. It is often drunk in a social environment of friends and family, which is healthful.[3]

Wine Labels Tout Health Benefits, Sort Of

These days, the government is allowing wine makers to advertise that wine may be good for you. But the wording is very evasive. The label reads, "The proud people who made this wine encourage you to consult your family doctor about the health effects of wine consumption." This is a hint that, for some folks, wine may be healthful.

But alcohol is not perfect. I remember what it was like when I was a teenager with parents who were alcoholics . . .

This was a far cry from the harmonious home of my early childhood. I saw firsthand how alcoholism could change people. My father, once so kind and caring, now only critized me. Meanwhile, my mom, who had always wanted only the best for us, was now often too drunk to take care of herself, much less our family. Violent arguments usually took place at the dinner table. My mother would end up crying and retreat to bed with a book in one hand, a drink in the other, while my angry father left the house for hours.

That was twenty years ago, and today I still find myself with painful memories of that time.

I am hardly alone. There are more than 21 million adult children of

Sons of Alcoholics

It is no surprise that adult male children of alcoholics are more likely to become alcoholics than men raised in nonalcoholic families. Worse yet, alcoholism is not the only problem with which adult sons may contend.

According to experts, sons of alcoholics may fall victim to lack of self-esteem, relationship problems, and fears of inadequacy.

Building up self-confidence is a must for adult sons who want to find the road to recovery. Here are five tips for adult children of alcoholics: Break the silence; form healthy male relationships; find a mentor; seek spiritual guidance; and stop drinking if you have a problem.

alcoholics. According to the National Institute on Alcohol Abuse and Alcoholism, 14 million people abuse alcohol or are alcoholic. Of that number, more men than women are alcohol-dependent or have alcohol-related problems.

While red wine can be good for your health, it can also be harmful. Alcohol depletes nutrients zinc and magnesium in the body; it can up the number of free radicals in the body; it can cause liver damage; alcohol drunk by pregnant women can lead to low-birth babies with lower IQs; social drinking can progress into alcoholism; alcohol damages the brain; it impairs the function of the digestive tract; and it may up your risk of breast cancer.[4]

What's more, wine can pack on the fat, which is not heart-healthy. One 4-ounce glass packs 100 calories. That can add up. Also, if you're migraine-prone, it's best to stay clear of red wine, which is one culprit. And the American Cancer Society reports that alcohol can cause serious liver damage.

Sadly enough, I know this can be true. At 74, my father became ill. I can tell you from my heart that it was the most painful ordeal he and I have ever experienced. My dad was in great physical pain for weeks. He died on February 28, 1998. On his certificate of death it reads: *Immediate cause: liver failure; Due to: liver abscess; Due to: liver cancer.* And to this day, since alcoholism runs in my family, I have never drank alcohol—not a sip.

THE ALTERNATIVES TO RED WINE FOR HEALTH

If you are drinking red wine for health benefits, think twice. "There are less toxic ways to get the benefits of the antioxidants, polyphenols, and other substances found in red wine," says Crayhon. "Fruits, veg-

Grape Juice Works Like Wine

One study at the University of Wisconsin Medical school, led by John D. Folts, reveals that three glasses of purple grape juice equal the blood-clotting stopping power of a glass of wine. He believes that it's the flavonoids, not the alcohol, that help ward off heart attacks among people who drink red wine.

etables, garlic, spices, herbs, and supplements can give you just as much antioxidant benefit if not more." And so can red wine vinegar.[5]

And now red wine vinegar, like grape juice, is being considered as a tradeoff for red wine. "Actually, red wine vinegar is just red wine that has soured," says Dr. Mindell. And does he believe it has any resveratrol in it? "Yes! It's a healthy thing to use."

Healthy indeed. As a nondrinker, I'm hardly alone. In fact, Dr. Magaziner admits that he is not a big drinker. He said to me, "I'm like you—I just don't enjoy alcohol. But I do eat a lot of red grapes." And I consume red grapes, grape juice, and red wine vinegar for the nonalcoholic protection.

UC Davis Enologist Turns Wine to Vinegar

Imagine this: You're the department winemaker and cellar master at the University of California–Davis department of viticulture and enology. The wine they produce is for research—not to drink or sell. So, when a study is done, rather than toss the good stuff out, it's put in a vinegar barrel. Ernie Farinias does just that.

Farinias, like other small-time vinegar makers (Chef Sal Campagna creates his vinegar, too), insists that it's easy to do—and he's been making homemade red wine vinegar for more than a quarter of a century.

If you have leftover red or dry white wine, get a vinegar barrel (a 1-gallon glass jar will do) and wash it well. Then, round up mother of vinegar (available in some wine specialty shops) and distilled water. Mix the mother with the wine in your clean container. Add one part water to three parts wine. It will dilute the wine and "cut the alcohol"—according to Farinias. Cover the container with cheesecloth and secure with a rubber band. Let it sit at room temperature for about two to three weeks. Then, siphon the vinegar out of its container and pour into a clean bottle with a metallic lid.

Want more vinegar? Put this new batch in a clean 5-gallon oak barrel. Each time you have leftover wine, dilute it just like you did before. But use caution, nutritionists say homemade vinegar is unpredictable and should never be used for canning or preserving—for safety's sake.[6]

Important Healing Hints to Remember

✓ Red wine vinegar contains polyphenols—and maybe resveratrol.
✓ Red wine vinegar is fat-free.
✓ You can add red wine vinegar to fruits and vegetables and get additional antioxidants.
✓ Red wine vinegar does not cause liver damage.

CHAPTER

9

Is Red Wine Vinegar Good for You?

The bitterer the salad of endives, the stronger must be the vinegar.

—Palestinian Proverb[1]

Not only are red wine vinegar's specific nutrients good for preventing health ailments but it can help treat disease, too. Many health practitioners emphasize its antioxidant vitamins, which can help you stave off age-related diseases and keep you living a longer, healthier life, too.

But there is *sooo* much more to know about the hidden ingredients in red wine. Here are expert reports and anecdotes about red wine vinegar (and a few of my own experiences) to show you how this condiment, like apple cider vinegar, is a gold mine.

Red Wine Vinegar and Heart Disease

The frightening fact is, heart disease, not cancer, is the Number 1 killer of both men—and women—in the United States. According to the American Heart Association, over half a million women will die of heart disease, stroke, or other cardiovascular disease in 1999. One out of five women have some form of cardiovascular disease.

Some risk factors for heart disease include high blood pressure, high cholesterol and a high-fat diet, and obesity. But don't despair. Red wine vinegar comes to the rescue.

For one, flavonoid-rich like wine, vinegar may help lower your total cholesterol level and prevent the oxidation of LDL cholesterol, the "bad" cholesterol, says Allan Magaziner, D.O. Translation: less risk of heart attacks and strokes.

Danish researchers found that weekly consumption of wine may cut stroke. In a 16-year study of 13,329 people, those who said they drank wine on a weekly basis—about one to six glasses per week—had a 34 percent lower risk of stroke than those who never or hardly ever drank wine. Those who said they had wine daily had a 32 percent reduction in risk. Those who drank beer or spirits did not have a significant reduction in stroke risk.[2]

One reason for wine's protective effects, the researchers say, may be its flavonoids and tannins—nutrients that may help inhibit the plaque obstructions that cause heart attacks and strokes.[3]

But note, the American Heart Association does not recommend that you start drinking to reduce your risk of heart disease and stroke. Research shows there is a higher risk of heart disease linked with drinking too much alcohol.[4] (My mother was taking blood pressure medication in between drinking bourbon and water.) Also, if red wine vinegar does, in fact, contain resveratrol like red wine—and doctors and researchers believe that it may—it can fight heart disease, too. How exactly does red wine work?

Research at the University of Illinois, conducted by Dr. John Pezzuto, shows intriguing data about resveratrol. "First, it inhibits the formation of blood clots, which can trigger both heart attack and stroke. Second, it plays a role in cholesterol metabolism, which may prevent the formation of artery-clogging plaque," reports Dr. Earl Mindell.[5]

Another way to stave off heart disease is by eating a low-fat diet. "Eating a balanced diet where less than 30 percent of the calories come from fat is very important," said Rebecca Reeves, a Baylor assistant professor of medicine. "Whole grain cereals, pasta products, and at least five servings of fruit and vegetables a day will help women maintain a healthy weight." And red wine vinegar can help flavor many of these heart-healthy foods.

Keep in mind, red wine vinegar is used in low-fat, hearty-healthy dishes such as salads, pasta plates, vegetables, and beans. In fact, beans are full of heart-healthy soluble fiber—the kind that helps control blood fat levels. James Anderson, M.D., a researcher based in Lexington, Kentucky, has found that eating just one cup of cooked dried beans a day can reduce artery-clogging LDL, the "bad" cholesterol, by 20 percent.

And our recipes at the end of this book include nutritious beans teamed with health-boosting red wine vinegar. This, in turn, can give you good nutrition such as you'll find at the Pritikin Longevity Center in Santa Monica, California.

Pritikin's director of nutrition services, Susan Massaron, says they do indeed include low-sodium vinegar (red wine, balsamic, and rice) in their meal plans. Why? "We use it as a seasoning," she says.

"Since our participants are on a low-sodium eating program, we try to keep our sodium very, very low. We find that the acidity from the vinegar gives an underlying sharpness to the food. It gives an edge to the food that substitutes very nicely for salt. It gives the illusion of salt without actually adding the sodium," adds Massaron. And note, Pritikin does not use seasoned vinegars because of the sodium content.

Why is it so important to have a low-sodium diet? "Primarily what we're keeping the sodium low for is to ward off hypertension or to correct hypertension or high blood pressure," says Massaron. Plus, for many people, she adds, by reducing their sodium intake, they will significantly reduce their blood pressure.

I remember when I was in college, my diet lacked nutrient-rich, low-fat foods. In fact, while I had classes scheduled back to back, I didn't allow myself a chance to eat a proper diet. I was living on diet soda and sunflower seeds. Then, one day I took my blood pressure at one of those self-service tests at drugstores. It was 150/90! I was shocked. I immediately stopped my high-salt diet. And in no time my blood pressure was back to a healthy 120/80.

Red Wine Vinegar and Cancer

Another benefit of red wine vinegar is its flavonoids, which can help guard against cancer. "Most of the studies performed on flavonoids have demonstrated their effectiveness in the prevention and treatment of various cancers. Some of the compounds that display antitumor effects are quercetin, hesperidin, genistein, rutin, naringin, catechin, and Pycnogenol®," reports Dr. Magaziner. And red wine vinegar may contain many if not all of these disease-fighting compounds.[6]

Research suggests that resveratrol inhibits the development of cancer in animals as well as prevents the progression of cancer. However, the jury is still out on how effective resveratrol is as an anticancer compound since human research is still needed in this area.

Another big benefit of flavonoid-rich red wine vinegar: paired with vegetables and fruits high in antioxidant vitamins C, E, and beta-carotene, you can prevent a number of cancers. These vitamins trap the free-radical molecules that cause normal cells to become cancerous. According to the American Cancer Society, studies show that a diet high in vegetables can lower cancer risk.

In addition, munching on more veggies and fruits and eating less meat may help stave off breast cancer, according to a past study. Researchers examined a link between intake of meats, vegetables, and fruits with levels of oxidative DNA damage in 21 healthy women (who had a high risk because they had a close relative with breast cancer) while consuming their usual diet or a diet low in fat.

"Everyone has damaged DNA from which cancer can potentially develop. The question is whether a healthier diet can reduce or repair the damaged DNA levels," says Cyndi Thomson, R.D., American Dietetic Association spokesperson and researcher at the University of Arizona's Cancer Center in Tucson. "And this study shows that eating more vegetables and fruits while eating meats in moderation has a positive effect."

Follow the ACS's guidelines to eat five or more servings of fruits and vegetables a day—especially vegetables from the cabbage family, such as broccoli, cauliflower, and Brussels sprouts. Studies show that phytochemicals (found only in plant foods) known as indole-3-carbinols found in cruciferous vegetables help to lower estrogen-causing cancer.

Plus, beans are superhealthy for you too. Beans also contain many compounds, such as phytoestrogens, phytates, and isoflavones, that are believed to have cancer-fighting properties. In fact, studies have shown that a diet rich in beans can reduce the risk of breast, lung, and pancreatic cancer. Try our Five-Bean Salad, which is teamed with red wine vinegar to help you get back on the healthy, five-a-day track.

Cancer-Fighting Vegetables

A diet high in a variety of nutrient-rich vegetables teamed with red wine vinegar may help prevent certain cancers. Here is a look at popular vegetables and the protection they may offer:

Super Food	Cancer-Fighting Substances	Protection For
Artichokes	Vitamin C, an antioxidant that stimulates tumor-attacking cells	Stomach, esophagus, larynx
Asparagus	Vitamin C and carotene, shown to fight cancer tumors by boosting white blood cell activity; selenium, a nutrient that activates infection fighting cells	Stomach, larynx, esophagus, lungs
Bell peppers	Vitamin C	Stomach, larynx, esophagus
Broccoli	Quercetin, an antioxidant that stimulates tumor-fighting cells; indoles-3-carbinol, a chemical that helps prevent "bad" estrogen that causes cancerous mutation in cells; and vitamin C	Lungs, colon, breasts
Corn	Protease inhibitors, which, according to research, may be potent cancer fighters	Breasts, colon
Green beans	Fiber, which may help decrease levels of cancer-promoting "bad" estrogen by escorting estrogen-contributing dietary fats out of the system	Breasts, colon
Salad greens	Beta-carotene, which may boost white blood cells; vitamin C	Stomach, larynx, esophagus
Tomato	Lycopene, an anticancer agent that helps destroy free radicals	Stomach, colon, mouth, throat

Red Wine Vinegar and Body Fat

Dr. McBarron knows firsthand about fat-fighting red wine vinegar. She usually eats low-fat fare. Is red wine vinegar a typical condiment on her dinner table? Yes, she says. From salads to main dishes, she can count on red wine vinegar to help maintain her weight and keep her body fat in check.

"Any time we cook chicken or fish, we usually use red wine vinegar. I sauté the vegetables in it." She will also add a couple of tablespoons of red wine vinegar when a recipe calls for a liquid.

"I'm married to an Italian. He grew up having pasta seven days a week. We always have pasta on the table. I'll have it four to five times a week. My husband is extremely healthy. He was raised on a healthy diet. When I met him I always did the salad dressing on the side because I was trying to watch my weight. And he always had oil and vinegar. I thought, 'Oh, that sounds terrible.' I don't even have salad dressing in my house anymore—it's always oil and vinegar for the taste and nutrients in it."

Dr. McBarron's One-Day Sample Vinegar Meal Plan

With the aid of Terri Brownlee, R.D., we designed a typical daily meal plan based on what works for Jan McBarron:

Breakfast

Fiber-Rich Fruit Salad: Mix ¼ cup each sliced strawberries, cantaloupe balls, grapes, and blueberries. Sprinkle with 1 tbsp organic mango vinegar.
1 cinnamon-raisin bagel
½ cup skim milk

Lunch

Slimming Stuffed Tomato: Stuff 1 medium tomato, hollowed, with ¼ cup each diced cucumber, green pepper, red onion, and cooked rice, and 1 tsp each olive oil and red wine vinegar. Broil 5–8 minutes.
½ wheat pita, toasted
1 cup honeydew or cantaloupe, cubed

Dinner

Tangy Chicken Bake: Bake 3 oz. skinless chicken breast topped with 1 tbsp each orange marmalade and raspberry or apple cider vinegar at 350° for 25 minutes.
½ cup wild rice
8 asparagus spears, steamed
½ cup mandarin oranges
Snacks: plenty of fresh fruit: blueberries, grapes, pears, and strawberries.

Losing Your Body Fat

Obesity is a major nutrition problem in the United States. According to the National Institutes of Health, more than 50 percent of all adults are overweight and a third are obese, and as many as 20 percent of children are obese.

While some body fat (the yellow stuff that insulates our bodies) is "good," too much of it is "bad." Says Tony Perrone, Ph.D., who is well known throughout Hollywood for creating lean bodies, "Body fat makes you pudgy and hides the definition of your muscles. It tends to sag in areas that are unsightly."

Worse, too much fat can cause a host of health problems. Excess body fat puts you at higher risk for diabetes, high blood pressure, heart disease, and stroke.

Again, red wine vinegar is one solution to taking and keeping fat off. "Vinegar is an allowable free food," says Dr. Perrone, "because it doesn't contribute any significant caloric intake. It doesn't harm a person's efforts to lose body fat."

So go ahead—switch to noncaloric, fat-free red wine vinegar salad dressing. When you toss a salad of mixed greens, substitute 2 tablespoons fat-free red wine vinegar for the 2 tablespoons of regular dressing you normally use three times a week. Calories saved per week: 420. Fat grams saved: 60. Your weight loss in one year: 6¼ lbs.

Fat-Fighting Red Wine Vinegar

Fat Dressing (1 Tbs)	Lean Dressing	Calories Saved
French dressing, low-cal	Red wine vinegar	15
French dressing, regular	Red wine vinegar	65
Mayonnaise	Red wine vinegar	100
1000-Island Dressing, regular	Red wine vinegar	80

I have witnessed people at a salad bar load up their plate with healthy, fresh vegetables and fruits. Then, they top it off with ladles of high-fat salad dressing (also high in preservatives, chemicals, and sodium). By doing this, you turn "good food into a high-fat food," says Massaron.

"If you are substituting red wine vinegar for a high-fat dressing," adds Massaron, "most definitely it would make a difference. A difference in your caloric and fat intake." In other words, lose the high-fat dressing and you'll lose the fat.

Longevity

So how does fat-fighting red wine vinegar help add years to your life anyhow? "Because of its antioxidant effects," answers Dr. Magaziner. "Any foods that have antioxidants in them are foods that we should incorporate into our diet because they help enhance our immune system. In turn, it helps us to feel healthier and hopefully reduce some of the diseases that we face as we get older."

When you eat a variety of foods that contain disease-fighting antioxidants, you can stall or prevent ailments associated with aging, adds Jeffrey Blumberg, Ph.D., associate director of the U.S. Department of Agriculture's Human Nutrition Research Center on Aging at Tufts University.

"You still get older," says Dr. Blumberg, "but you'll increase your lifespan." Medical doctors agree: the healthier you are, the younger your body stays. So go ahead—it's never too late to put these eight healthy, low-fat, antiaging foods teamed with age-fighting red wine vinegar on your menu! Just turn to our recipes in the back of this book.

Seven Antiaging Foods + RWV to Fight Father Time

1. **Carrots:** Beta-carotene-rich carrots keep your vision clear and sharp, according to studies at the USDA Human Nutrition Center on Aging in Boston.
2. **Red pepper:** Peppers, especially the red ones, are a great source of vitamin C and can enhance the body's immune function to help keep you healthy.
3. **Broccoli:** According to the American Cancer Society, studies show vegetables in the cabbage family (or crucifers) appear to protect against stomach and colon cancers. Eat more broccoli and cauliflower.
4. **Spinach:** Leafy green vegetables, which are rich in vitamin A and iron, can help keep your nails strong and healthy.
5. **Asparagus:** Low-cal asparagus is a good source of vitamin C, which works as an anti-inflammatory agent and can help fight arthritis aches and pains.
6. **Tofu:** According to the American Cancer Society, tofu can inhibit the type of estrogen that causes breast, uterine, and ovarian cancers.
7. **Fish:** Because it contains vital omega-3 fatty acids, fish can retard the aging process.

Not only is red wine vinegar plentiful with antiaging antioxidants, it's cholesterol free, sodium free, and fat free. And that without a doubt can help stave off age-related ailments such as heart disease and cancer, too.

IMPORTANT HEALING HINTS TO REMEMBER

✓ Red wine vinegar contains flavonoids (and perhaps heart-healthy resveratrol), which can help prevent high blood pressure, stroke, and heart attack.

✓ Red wine vinegar is rich in cancer-fighting antioxidants that can help lower cancer risk.

✓ Teamed with antioxidant-rich vegetables, red wine vinegar can help fight cancer.

✓ Red wine vinegar, which is low-cal, sodium free and fat-free can help you keep your body fat ratio lower.

✓ Red wine vinegar—which is free of cholesterol and sodium and fat—can help add years to your life.

✓ Plus, if you pair red wine vinegar with disease-fighting, antiaging foods, you can boost longevity.

PART 4

Other Natural Vinegars

CHAPTER

10

Healthy Rice Vinegar

Pure rice vinegar is the best among vinegar.[1]
—Togo Kuroiwa

For more than 3,000 years, the Chinese have been making rice vinegar. Rice vinegars come in red, white, brown, or black. They are most often used in Asian recipes that require vinegar.

The Japanese have been making vinegar since yesteryear, using rice as its basic material and utilizing the production method brought from ancient China. Yet new kinds of vinegar emerged in the 1910s in Japan. They were made of alcohol and petroleum and upstaged the traditional natural vinegar.

Rice Vinegar Is Diet-Friendly

Personally, I wasn't aware of rice vinegar until recently. My girlfriend, a good cook, is from Taiwan. One day when I was visiting her, she was making dinner. I was surprised that she used brown rice vinegar in the soup, salad, and fish. "It is no big deal," she said. It is a staple of her Asian diet.

Rice-wine vinegar is less acidic than other types, so you can use more of it in a vinaigrette with oil. That reduces both the grams of fat and the calories per serving. They are good for flavoring with herbs. And rice vinegar contains healthful ingredients. After all, it's made from rice.

Good Grains

In the 1940s the nutritional value of rice became popular thanks to Duke University's William Kempner, M.D., who created the Rice Diet to reduce high blood pressure. He believed that the low-sodium content of the rice and fruit had a good effect on blood pressure. Brown rice is also healthful because it provides fiber, plus 5 grams of protein per cup. It also has some vitamin E, and is high in selenium.

While rice vinegar, unlike apple cider and red wine vinegars, is not high in potassium, it is higher in phosphorus and calcium—two minerals your body needs. Although it has only trace elements of vitamins A, C, riboflavin, and niacin, rice vinegar does contain other ingredients, according to a national vinegar manufacturer.[2] Per 3½ ounces:

- Carbohydrates: 3 grams
- Calcium: 1 gram
- Sodium: 5 milligrams
- Potassium: 8 milligrams
- Phosphorous: 1 milligram

But it's not just the labeled ingredients in rice vinegar that make it healthful. It's the amino acids in vinegar that are the secret of pure rice vinegar's good-for-you healing power.

AMINO ACIDS: THE REAL ESSENCE OF RICE VINEGAR

When genuine natural rice vinegar is manufactured according to the method of production available from ancient times, it will contain more amino acids than any other vinegar.

Because of the amino acids in it, natural rice vinegar is an effective healer as well as a seasoning, according to *Rice Vinegar*'s author Togo Kuroiwa.[3]

According to the Japan Food Research Laboratories, pure rice vinegar contains many of the essential amino acids, which include lysine, histidine, alginine, valine, isoleucine, leucine, and phenylalanine.[4]

Remember how acidity and strong alkali are what originate a disease and the affected region always indicates strong alkali? If pure rice vinegar is rich in amino acids, which Kuroiwa believes it is, then it can neutralize alkali in the ailing body part.[5]

"Amino acid," he adds, "therefore, is the thing itself for curing disease and injury and showing great effect on the human body. As a result, we understand very well the various effects of vinegar which have been proven in the experiences gained by so many people over so many years since ancient times."[6]

While nutritionists agree that vinegar boasts amino acids—we don't know which ones are in rice vinegar. "Rice does have protein in it. So it would have amino acids in it. But the key is, how much rice is in the vinegar," says Connie Diekman, R.D. And nobody knows the quantity.

Rice vinegar is going to add to your daily required intake of amino acids. "The big question mark is," adds Diekman, "protein is digested in acid. So are we losing the amino acids because of the acidity of the vinegar?"

Herbal vinegar writer Maggie Oster adds, "Because the grain remains present throughout the fermentation and vinegar-producing process, this rice vinegar has a significant amino acid content. The medical claims made for Japanese rice vinegar include the ability to neutralize lactic acid in the body, alkalinize the blood, and generally promote good health."[7]

Rice Vinegar Success Stories

In his book, Kuroiwa provides various real people who reveal exactly how rice vinegar worked wonders.[8]

Jyosuke's Story: "Good for Broken Bone"

"It seems to me that rice vinegar is good for dislocation of bones and sprains. This is a case of a broken bone.

"My brother-in-law called on our home after getting a diagnosis from his doctor that he had a crack in his shoulder blade. He complained of not being able to lift his shoulder and claimed he had a high temperature.

"I had then heard of how good rice vinegar was for such a case. I decided to give him a rice vinegar wet dressing. I used about 0.3 pints of wheat flour to knead it with a wine cupful of vinegar and water and applied it all to the affected region.

"He said he felt very well and had no shoulder ache that night. He had a good night's sleep because of the wet dressing. He found the packing sheet completely dry the following morning. He changed it two or three times since then and found himself in good condition in his shoulder."

Kazuko's Story: "Good for Constipation"

After a stomach operation this woman suffered from lack of bowel movements. While someone told her that fasting was a solution, she decided to try rice vinegar enemas instead.

"I gave rice vinegar injections into the bowels three times a day—morning, midway and evening. I did that everytime I had a bath. On the third day after I started giving myself rice vinegar injections, I had a bowel movement . . . Three times a day, I had rice vinegar, each time sipping one wine cup full of it. I poured four or five tea cups full of rice vinegar into the bathtub and took a bath three times a day. After I had easy bowel movements."

Shizue's Story: "Good for Rhinitis"

"I heard that rice vinegar was good for rhinitis (inflammation of the nasal mucous membranes), and I thought I should try it. First, I had a tablespoon of vinegar in a cleaning device and cleaned my nose. I did this twice or I used 10cc of rice vinegar.

"I repeated this for three months. The mucous in my nose began to disappear. At the same time, I felt very good after cleansing the nose. Previously, if I didn't clean my nose for a week, I would have had a hard time with my nose closed up. Now, the nose stays the same even if I didn't wash my nose.

"It has been about a year since I started using vinegar. I cleanse my nose at least once a week. I feel wonderful and feel as if I have finally cured my nose. For your information, I think the amount of rice vinegar I use for cleaning my nose is just about right for me."

Important Healing Hints to Remember

✓ Amino acid–rich rice vinegar helps to balance the pH in the body.
✓ Rice vinegar can help fight aches, congestion, and constipation.
✓ Rice vinegar is a good flavoring with herbs in nutrient-dense foods.
✓ Rice vinegar users believe it really works.

CHAPTER

11

The Balsamic Vinegar Boom

This vinegar tastes like it's got oil in it![1]
—Richard Simmons

For 1,000 years, balsamic vinegar coined "Aceto Balsamico" has been considered for its medicinal properties.

In the seventeenth century, people used it as a gargle, tonic, and air purifier against the plague. The word "Balsamico" in Italian means balm, which connotes a healing, soothing medicine. And it was.

In the twenty-first century, the belief that balsamic vinegar is nature's miracle worker still remains. Today, it is very popular both in Europe and the United States. However, many people are clueless as to why it is so good. They just know it is.

An Italian Thing

Balsamic vinegar is traditionally made in Modena, Italy, and historically made from Trebbiano grapes grown around the hills of Modena. The grapes are allowed to ripen until they are supersweet before harvest time. The juice is then filtered and poured into a progression of casks made from a variety of woods—such as oak, chestnut, ash, cherry, and mulberry, from which it reaps a deep reddish-brown color.

Vinegar that gets the grade "traditional vecchio" is aged at least 12 years, while the variety called "tradizionale extra vecchio" is aged at least 25 years—and can cost more than $100 per bottle.

"In Modena, balsamic vinegar is not just vinegar, it is a symbol of sophistication, a good investment, and a way of life. The prices range from a few dollars per bottle to more than $300 for a 7½ ounce bottle from a batteria dated 1730. This makes vinegar a very extravagant and pricey condiment," reports vinegarman Lawrence Diggs.

"In Italy, it is so highly prized that sometimes it is not sold at all. It is saved by the family for special gifts for dowries. The very best balsamics may be reserved for close associates and family," adds Diggs.

Balsamic vinegar as a treasured gift? Absolutely, says chef Sal Campagna, who is of Italian descent. His parents were born in Sicily. And for their seventy-fifth wedding anniversary, Sal turned to balsamic vinegar. It's true. A bottle from Modena (priced at $120 for 8 ounces) was part of the anniversary dinner package. At his restaurant, Salvatores, which specializes in Continental cuisine, he provided an extravagant celebration dinner. For dessert, the creative chef drizzled the rich vinegar over vanilla ice cream for forty people.

What's more, when he told me this story, I just had to indulge. After my dinner at Salvatore's (salad with red wine vinegar and olive oil dressing, salmon, and a baked potato), I indulged in the balsamic vinegar decadent delight. And to my surprise, the Italian dessert was *magnifico!*

The two kinds of balsamic vinegar are the real stuff *(Aceto Balsamico naturale)*, like the vinegar I had at Salvatores, and the industrial or imitation. The industrial version is boiled-down Trebbiano grapes that have been mixed with regular vinegar, then flavored and colored with carmelized sugar, herbs, and other ingredients. It is aged about a year.

Bob Rubinelli, founder of Rubinelli, Inc., in Cicero, Illinois, explained it to me, which has a more Italian flavor to it: "I traveled to Modena, Italy, to find out firsthand about balsamic vinegar. My hosts were two local producers, Mr. Aggazzotti and Mr. Galletti, who graciously took me through the entire production process at their acetificio and explained to me the two basic types of vinegar.

"First there is 'Traditional Balsamic Vinegar of Modena.'" He wasn't disappointed to see the legend of this product, dating back nearly 1,000 years. He passionately raves about the Trebbiano grapes, transferring the unfermented juice to wooden barrels, and the forever-long aging process.

"The second balsamic vinegar product is the commercial/industrial version. This is the version we so commonly see on the grocery store shelves. It is an imitation produced by adding sugar and flavoring to a small amount of strong wine vinegar," he explains. "It is an affordable, versatile, delicious vinegar that imparts some of the same characteristics of the traditional and is the basis for a fine salad dressing, marinade, or cooking ingredient. This commercial balsamic vinegar sells for under four dollars per seventeen-ounce bottle."

Adds Rubinelli: "There is a third type of balsamic vinegar that will vary according to the producer—this is a blend of traditional and commercial. Aggazzotti, for example, produces a product that is five percent traditional and costs under $10."[2]

The fact remains, balsamic vinegar—real and imitation—has soared in its popularity due to the American discovery in the 1970s and 1980s. But just how nutritious is it anyhow?

Good Stuff

Not everybody is going to buy the expensive balsamic vinegar. A lot of folks will, however, purchase balsamic vinegar at specialty shops or health food stores. And that's where you can get a bottle of organic balsamic vinegar. On the front label (such as Spectrum Naturals) it will read: "Product of Modena, Italy. Produced in wooden casks. No added sulfites." Sounds good to me.

Then, turn that balsamic vinegar bottle around and you'll be greeted by this: "Following centuries of Italian tradition our Organic Balsamic Vinegar is carefully blended from grape must and wine from Trebbiano and Lambrisco grapes. Produced in wood, the result is a richly flavored vinegar with intense aromas and delicately balanced sweet and sour taste."

Nutrition Facts
No added sugar, sulfites, or artificial colorings
Serving Size 1

Calories	6
Calories from fat	0
Total Fat	0 g
Total Carbohydrate	2 g
Sugars	2 g
Total Protein	0 g

Not a significant source of cholesterol, dietary fiber, vitamin A, vitamin C, calcium, and iron.

Ingredients: Organically grown and processed wine vinegar and organic concentrated grape must.

(*Source:* Spectrum Naturals.)

So what happens if you check out a bigger quantity of balsamic vinegar. One national vinegar production company did just that.[3] Here's what you get for 3½ ounces, or almost a half cup:

- Calcium: 12 grams
- Carbohydrates: 30 grams
- Fat: 0
- Sodium: 20 milligrams
- Potassium: 70 milligrams
- Sugars: 30 grams
- Phosphorous: 20 milligrams

It also has trace elements of ash, vitamin A, thiamine, riboflavin, niacin, iron, and vitamin C. But there's more to it.

SECRET INGREDIENTS

As with red wine vinegar, the labeled contents aren't the entire story. Balsamic vinegar, like its grape-filled counterpart, contains powerful antioxidants that protect against heart disease by blocking the oxidation LDL—the "bad" cholesterol—and may even fight cancer.

Recently, upon my request and interest, Dr. Leroy Creasy analyzed a bottle of his personal balsamic vinegar. Indeed, like other wine vinegars, it was high in polyphenol activity, he reported. More scientific research is required before we know just how potent balsamic vinegar is in fighting disease.

THE BALSAMIC BANDWAGON

Meanwhile, Italian restaurants use it. Celebrities use it. Doctors use it. And even health spas use this dark vinegar with a mellow, slightly syrupy taste.

Richard Simmons, a well-known fitness expert, says balsamic vinegar is one of his Top 10 favorite foods. "I love salads, but most fat free dressings aren't palate-pleasing. This vinegar tastes like it's got oil on it! I use it on salads or to marinate. I've even used it in casseroles."[4]

BALSAMIC VINEGAR AND OLIVE OIL

Is balsamic vinegar and olive oil a good and healthy mix? "Olive oil provides your monounsaturated fatty acids. So if you're looking for a salad dressing option—it's wonderful," says Connie Diekman, R.D. "The major thing that I hear from people is that the flavor combination is so full it almost feels decadent."

Chef Campagna told me that he used to plan menus for San Francisco's World Champion 49ers and their former coach, Bill Walsh. Often, the salad dressing of choice would include balsamic vinegar. Balsamic vinaigrette was their favorite dressing, and Sal would use different ratios of olive oil.

If you marry balsamic vinegar and olive oil, does it make a pleasant and healthy mix? Absolutely, say chefs, nutritionists, and doctors. Not only will you get the cancer-fighting, antioxidant-rich polyphenols in vinegar, but heart-healthy monounsaturated olive oil that forms its base in a vinaigrette can help to lower your cholesterol levels, too. (See Chapter 13, "Combining Vinegars and Garlic, Onions and Olive Oil.")

Balsamic Vinaigrette

❖ ❖ ❖

¼ cup balasmic vinegar
6 tablespoons water
1 tablespoon Dijon mustard
1 tablespoon freshly ground black pepper
½ teaspoon minced dried basil
2 tablespoons olive oil (or canola oil)

In a small mixing bowl, whisk together balsamic vinegar, water, Dijon mustard, black pepper, and dried basil. Vigorously whisk in a thin stream of olive oil. Store vinaigrette in refrigerator until ready to use. Will keep up to 2 weeks in the refrigerator. Serves 12. *Health perks:* 23 calories per tablespoon; 2 g total fat; 0 cholesterol; 6 IU vitamin A; 32 mg sodium.

(*Source:* Chef Michel Stroot of the Golden Door Spa.)

Good Eating Vinaigrette Tips

- Add seasonings a little at a time; taste and add more if needed.
- Make seasoned vinaigrette ahead of time to allow flavors to marry.
- To use less oil and still have a vinaigrette with body, get out the blender. Reduce the amount of oil by 2–3 tablespoons; add 2–3 tablespoons water. Blend on high 1 full minute to emulsify the vinegar and water in the oil.
- Dress a leafy green salad lightly! Let the flavors of the greens shine through.
- For pasta, rice, and potato salads, use a little more wine vinegar and less oil in the vinaigrette. These salads are invigorated by the flavor of tangy wine vinegar and can get by with less oil.

(Source: Four Monks: Nakano.)

MORE COMMON VINEGARS, PLEASE

- *Sherry vinegar:* Derived from the southwest region of Spain, sherry vinegars are made like balsamics. They're aged for several years before bottling and cost more, too.
- *Malt vinegar:* From Europe's beer breweries comes malt vinegar, which is made from fermented malted barley. It's especially "in" in England, the place where it's "in" to sprinkle it on fish and chips. In fact, these days you can even buy potato chips that contain malt vinegar.
- *Ume plum vinegar:* Ume plum vinegar comes from what else? Ume boshi plums. Since it is made with salt, you can add less salt to your foods.
- *Distilled white vinegar*: White vinegar is praised for its versatile household uses, from washing windows to cleaning a coffee maker. Unlike apple cider vinegar, which boasts 240 milligrams of potassium, distilled white vinegar has a mere 36 milligrams of this mineral.

IMPORTANT HEALING HINTS TO REMEMBER

✓ Balsamic vinegar is high in antioxidant polyphenols.
✓ Balsamic vinegar is fat-free.
✓ Balsamic vinegar is high potassium.
✓ Balsamic vinegar is tasty.
✓ Balsamic vinegar and olive oil are the dressing of the new millennium.

CHAPTER

12

Healing Herbal Vinegars

From sublime sage and majoram to zesty jalapeño garlic, flavored vinegars are a treat for both the palate and the eye.

—Heinz U.S.A.

Combine herbs, berries, flowers, and vinegar and what do you get? Healthful herbal or infused vinegars that can be an extra boon to your health, too.

Dioscorides, who reportedly traveled through Egypt with Nero's army, found that Egyptian medicines included vinegar combined with honey, brine, thyme, or squill, and this mixture was used for many health ailments.[1]

Like healing vinegar, herbs—such as parsley, sage, rosemary, and thyme—have been shown to contribute not only to good lyrics, thanks to Simon and Garfunkel, but to good health. You can make your own herbal vinegars and reap a host of therapeutic effects from these herbs mixed with wine, rice, or apple cider vinegar. Think about using some of these herbs steeped in vinegar for the therapeutic benefits you can obtain both outside and inside your body:

CHAMOMILE *(Anthemis nobilis):* Chamomile, a common folk medicinal herb, has been used to treat a variety of health ailments. The dried flowers brewed in a tea help combat gastrointestinal symptoms, minor infections, and skin disorders.

Recent research shows that chamomile contains apigenin, a flavonoid which has antioxidant properties and may inhibit skin tumor formation. Thus it could be beneficial in sunscreens.[2]

RED CLOVER *(Trifolium pratense):* This herb is phytoestrogen-rich, which is believed to be soothing and healing.

COMFREY *(Symphytum officinale):* The herb comfrey may aid in healing cuts and help soothe minor burns and swelling faster.

ECHINICEA *(Echinacea angustfolia):* This infection-fighting herb can help kill bacteria, fungi, viruses, and other germs. Echinicea contains a natural antibiotic called echinacoside and a germ-fighting compound called echinacein. It is also used externally for cuts, burns, and cold sores.

EUCALYPTUS *(Eucalyptus globulus):* This herb relieves runny noses and helps clear the sinuses and respiratory system. It's used in many saunas to help people breathe easy. I personally use fresh eucalyptus in my shower for the wonderful aroma. It also has antiseptic, antiviral, and decongestant benefits.

FENNEL *(Foeniculum vulgare):* Some mainstream doctors find that the use of herbs can treat everyday ailments. Fennel used in a tea has been known to relieve symptoms of abdominal discomfort, such as gas, bloating, and belching.

HORSETAIL *(Equisetum arvense):* Both the American Indians and the Chinese use silicon-containing horsetail to stop bleeding and to help wounds and broken bones heal faster. It's the solubility of silica in fluids of wounds or in the poultice materials, and its absorption directly into blood and cells at the site of the wound, that makes horsetail work, according to herb expert Daniel B. Mowrey, Ph.D.[3]

European research reveals that horsetail stops bleeding and helps build up the blood. It has good antibiotic action, too. "Silica acid, or horsetail tea," adds Dr. Mowrey, "causes a slight rise in white blood cell count, and thereby enhances nonspecific resistance to diseases of many types."[4]

JUNIPER *(Juniperus communis):* The dried fruit and leafy branches have been used as an antiseptic, and act as a diuretic. Also, juniper has been used as a detox and body cleanser, as well as for reducing muscle pain.

LAVENDER *(Lavandula angustifolia):* This fragrance is used in aromatherapy for relaxation. Also, you can drink lavender tea, which acts as a mild sedative. It is also used to help heal scars, minimize stretch marks, and soothe insect bites.

MINT (*Mentha spp.*): Mint is beneficial for normal skin, refreshes, and cools. Peppermint not only can soothe tense muscles, but can be used to cure an upset stomach.

NETTLE *(Urtica spp.):* To stave off allergies, congestion, watery eyes, and other hay fever symptoms, nettle may do the trick.

OREGANO *(Oregano vulgare):* Oregano oil is both antiseptic and anti-inflammatory. Not only does it kill bacteria, viruses, fungi, and other germs, it also fights infection, from colds to the flu. Also, oregano contains carvacrol, a type of phenol that is potent as an antiseptic.[5]

As an anti-inflammatory, oregano can be rubbed on aching muscles to relieve strains, and used externally to help heal burns and wounds, reports Dr. Mindell.[6]

PARSLEY *(Petroselinum crispum):* This cleansing herb is packed with disease-fighting antioxidant vitamins A, C, and E. Also, it boasts plenty of iron. Parsley gets its good reputation, however, for its diuretic action. Plus, it's believed to ease PMS symptoms, including cramps, hormonal mood swings, and bloating.

"Parsley does not allow salt to be reabsorbed into body tissues and literally forces debris out to the kidneys, liver and bladder. It is this ability which has saved lives—especially in cases where urine was backing up and poisoning the kidneys and liver," reports Laurel Dewey, an herbalist in Glenwood Springs, Colorado.[7]

ROSEMARY *(Rosmarinus officinalis):* This ancient therapeutic herb contains calcium, magnesium, sodium, and potassium, all of which help balance fluids surrounding nerves and heart tissues.

In fact, rosemary may help to lower blood pressure. The rosemary leaf may have other positive cardiovascular effects owing to its rosemaricine content, and the flavonoid pigment diosmin.

Rosemary may also be known as the cancer-fighting herb. A research project at Penn State proves this to be true and shows that rosemary could reduce the risk of cancer in rats given a powerful carcinogen.[8]

SAGE *(Salvia officinalis):* Herbalists claim sage is a natural astringent and antiseptic. It's recommended for gingivitis and to soothe a sore throat. But caution: pregnant women should not take it.

THYME *(Thymus vulgaris)*: Thyme is a delicate herb which is a natural source of iron, magnesium, silicon, sodium, and thiamine. Its power is as an antiseptic and a general healing tonic. It is believed to be helpful in cases of anemia. It can also subdue coughing relieve intestinal ailments.

Make Your Own Therapeutic Vinegar

Just start with dry whole herb sprigs—from thyme to rosemary. Place a couple of sprigs in a sterile pint jar. Heat two cups of vinegar to a simmer in a small stainless steel or ceramic saucepan. Pour the steeped vinegar into the jar (use a funnel) and allow to cool. Let stand for seven days before using. It's recommended to store it at room temperature.

CREATE YOUR OWN FLAVORED VINEGARS

You can make your own flavored vinegars by blending your favorite herbs, fruits, and spices. The following recipes are courtesy of Heinz.

- **Basil Garlic Vinegar:** Place ½ cup coarsely chopped basil leaves and 2 cloves peeled, split garlic in a sterilized pint jar. Heat Heinz Wine or Distilled White Vinegar to just below boiling point. Fill jar with vinegar and cap tightly. Allow to stand 3 to 4 weeks. Strain vinegar, discarding basil and garlic. Pour vinegar into a clean sterilized jar, adding fresh basil for garnish if desired. Seal tightly. Use in dressings for rice, pasta, antipasto salads, or in flavored mayonnaise.
- **Herb Vinegar**: Make a bouquet of 3 to 4 sprigs each parsley, sage, marjoram, and thyme, and place in a sterilized pint jar with ½

teaspoon whole black peppercorns. Heat Heinz Distilled White or Wine Vinegar to just below the boiling point. Fill jar with vinegar and cap tightly. Allow to stand 3 to 4 weeks. Strain vinegar, discarding herbs. Pour vinegar into a clean sterilized jar, adding sprigs of fresh herbs for garnish if desired. Seal tightly. Use in marinades for mushrooms or artichokes, or in dressing for tossed green or pasta salads.

- **Lemon Thyme Vinegar:** Remove peel (colored portion only) from 1 lemon in a thin spiral and place in a sterilized pint jar with 4 to 5 sprigs of thyme or lemon thyme. Heat Heinz Distilled White Vinegar to just below the boiling point. Fill jar with vinegar and cap tightly. Allow to stand 3 to 4 weeks. Strain vinegar, discarding peel and thyme. Pour vinegar into a clean sterilized jar, adding fresh thyme sprig and peel for garnish. Seal tightly. Use in dressings for tossed green salads or marinades for vegetables.
- **Jalapeño Garlic Vinegar:** Cut a few small slits in 2 small jalapeño peppers and place in a decorative bottle with 2 cloves peeled garlic. Heat Heinz Wine or Apple Cider Vinegar to just below the boiling point. Fill bottle with vinegar and cap tightly. Allow to stand 3 to 4 weeks. Use in dressing for taco, tomato and onion, or avocado salads, or when making salsa.

The Fruit-Flavored Vinegar Craze

Fruity vinegars boast health benefits, too, while adding a splash of flavor to meals. The fresh flavor of fruit vinegars—such as raspberry, blueberry, strawberry, and orange—can perk up a healthful salad or make a tasty marinande for poultry. Plus, antioxidant vitamin C in oranges, raspberries and blueberries enhance your immune system and keep disease at bay.

Blueberry Youth-Boosting Bliss

A new study reported by the National Institute on Aging, U.S. Department of Agriculture, shows that animals fed a blueberry extract diet, rich in naturally derived antioxidants, had fewer age-related motor changes and performed better than their counterparts on memory tests. In result, blueberries may guard the body against damage from oxidative stress—one of the biological processes linked to aging.[9] (See the recipes in Part 7 that include blueberry vinegar.)

- *Raspberry vinegar* is a very popular wine vinegar that's been infused with fresh raspberry. It has a stunning red color and taste like the berry. Raspberry vinegar is an acid syrup made with fruit juice, sugar, and white wine vinegar and, when added to water, forms an excellent cooling drink in summer, suitable also in feverish cases, where the acid is not an objection. It makes a useful gargle for sore throats.[10]
- *Strawberry vinegar* provides health benefits, too. Strawberry-infused vinegar, which uses balsamic vinegar, is a source of vitamins A and C, and is low in calories and free of fat, cholesterol, and sodium.
- *Mango honey vinegar* is sherry wine vinegar with mangoes added. This infused vinegar contains 6 mg of vitamin C, has a whopping 266 IU of vitamin A, and is fat and cholesterol free and has 23 calories and 1 mg of sodium per serving.

Try these fruit vinegars, and for your health's sake, enjoy:

Strawberry-Basil Balsamic Infusion

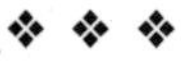

Very ripe strawberries, even soft, but not spoiled, make the most flavorful infusion. So don't toss those "tired" strawberries. Make an infusion!

3 cups balsamic vinegar
7½ ounces strawberries (1½ cups of trimmed, quartered strawberries)
1 cup packed fresh basil leaves
1 cup water

Push quartered strawberries into a sterilized 1-quart bottle or drop into sterilized 1-quart Mason jar. Roll up basil leaves and push into bottle or jar. Bring balsamic vinegar to a simmer in a medium-size saucepan. Remove from heat and add the water. Using a funnel, pour hot vinegar-water mixture into bottle. Set aside, allow to cool, then cover. Keep out on the counter overnight; refrigerate the next day. Makes 5 cups or forty 2-tablespoon servings.

(*Source:* Sous chef Josh Carroll of the Golden Door Spa.)

Mango Honey Vinegar

❖ ❖ ❖

1½ cups sherry wine vinegar
1½ cups fresh orange juice
½ cup honey
10 ounces ripe mangoes (1½ to 2 cups), peeled, small dice
2 teaspoons chili sauce, with garlic,
2–3 tablespoons fructose

In a medium-sized saucepan, bring sherry wine vinegar and orange juice to a boil. Stir in honey, mangoes, and chili sauce. Let cool. Push through fine sieve. Add fructose, if needed. Transfer to sterilized glass container. Keep refrigerated.

(*Source:* Chef Michel Stroot of the Golden Door Spa.)

Health Fact!

Food Safety Alert: It is difficult to determine the exact shelf life of homemade flavored vinegars which include oils. American Dietetic Association (ADA) nutritionists question the safety issue since we do not know if we can prevent food-borne illnesses.

According to the ADA, as many as 33 million Americans yearly contract food-borne illnesses. The home is a common place for food-borne illness to occur. But the ADA is constantly at work learning how consumers can protect themselves and their families from the threat of food-borne illness.

IMPORTANT HEALING HINTS TO REMEMBER

✓ Chamomile	For stomach ailments, minor infections, and skin disorders
✓ Red clover	Soothes, heals
✓ Comfrey	Heals cuts, burns, and swelling
✓ Echinacea	Antiseptic, heals
✓ Eucalyptus	Antiseptic, deodorant, stimulates, soothes, heals
✓ Fennel	Soothes abdominal woes
✓ Horsetail	Heals minor wounds, antibiotic
✓ Juniper	Relieves muscle soreness, cleansing
✓ Lavender	Sedative, soothes insect bites
✓ Mint	Treats normal skin, soothes tense muscles and tummy
✓ Nettle	Treats allergies, congestion
✓ Oregano	Antiseptic and anti-inflammatory, relieves muscle soreness, heals wounds
✓ Parsley	Cleansing
✓ Rosemary	Heart-healthy, cancer-fighting
✓ Sage	Astringent, antiseptic, soothes a sore throat
✓ Thyme	Antiseptic, helps anemia, coughs, intestinal upsets
✓ Raspberry	It can help soothe a sore throat

PART 5

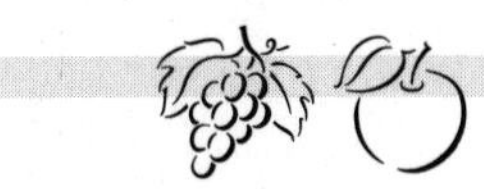

FUTURE VINEGAR

CHAPTER

13

Combining Vinegars and Garlic, Onions, and Olive Oil

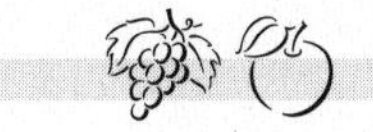

Our Garrick's a salad; for him we see
Oil, vinegar, sugar and saltiness agree.
—Oliver Goldsmith[1]

Vinegar is one of the oldest known ingredients used in cooking. And health-wise it can stand alone as a healthy condiment. But by teaming other superhealing foods—garlic, onions, and olive oil—with apple cider, red wine, balsamic, and rice vinegar you've added a powerful punch to any recipe.

In umpteen recipes you'll find vinegar paired with garlic, onions, and olive oil. It's common in the Mediterranean world and now in the United States, too. Not only do these extra vinegar ingredients help add flavor to food, but research continues to show that this trio can enhance your health—and boost longevity, too. All three—and vinegars—help fight heart disease, cancer, obesity, colds, aging, and much, much more.

Garlic and Vinegar

Garlic *(Allium sativum)* has been touted for its extra-special health properties, today and yesterday. It's hot stuff. For at least 3,000 years, garlic dubbed "the stinking rose," has been used medicinally.

Garlic has a long history. Louis Pasteur, bacteriologist, used it for its antibiotic effects. Albert Schweitzer treated dysentery. In World Wars I and II, the British military used it to control infection and gangrene. Pliny wrote that it cured tuberculosis. Hippocrates believed it eased the pain of stings and bites. And people in 1918 used it to fight off the flu epidemic.

Today, the therapeutic uses of garlic have been noted in more than 1,000 scientific studies. Garlic has been found to lower cholesterol and high blood pressure, as well as ward off infections and cancer.

And research shows garlic and vinegar provide super benefits to our health taken together or alone. Either way, this powerful duo enhance the immune system, prevent heart ailments, and much more.

Superpower Ingredients

Garlic is chock-full of healthful nutrients. Here, take a close-up look at one average clove of garlic, which the U.S. Department of Agriculture did:

- .01 mg B_1
- .004 mg B_2
- 1.4 mg calcium
- 1.5 carbohydrate
- .07 iron
- .02 niacin
- 10 mg phosphorus
- 26 mg potassium
- .31 g protein
- .9 mg sodium
- .75 mg vitamin C

It's these very compounds that fulfill the ancient Telugu proverb—"Garlic is as good as 10 mothers."[2] And it very well may be that garlic is that good and even better. Here's why.

Garlic vs. Cancer: For many years, the National Cancer Institute has been studying how common foods can help safeguard against cancer—and garlic figures are high on their list.

"It helps protect cells from cancer-causing agents," says John

Milner, Ph.D., a nutritionist at Pennsylvania State University. "You get both preventive and therapeutic benefits from garlic. It will slow the progression of an existing tumor cell and it will block the formation of tumor cells.

Garlic vs. Infection. Garlic contains allicin, which is a strong antibiotic. It is believed that eating garlic can help ward off colds, flu, and bronchitis. It may be the antioxidant mineral selenium in garlic that protects cells from damage and fights off disease and infection.

A study at Boston City Hospital found that allicin was effective against a wide variety of bacteria including salmonellas, streptococcus, and microbes that cause influenza and pneumonia.[3]

Garlic vs. Heart Disease. Like red wine vinegar, garlic can help lower cholesterol. Even better, garlic can raise good cholesterol (HDL, high-density lipoprotein), which fights hardening of the arteries, according to a variety of studies.

Medical experts say that the French eat plenty of heart-healthy garlic. "In fact, the beneficial side of their alcohol consumption may be its ability to help the body absorb more of the beneficial substances in garlic," reports nutritionist Robert Crayhon.[4]

Onions and Vinegar

For centuries, doctors, philosophers, and common folk have praised the onion *(Allium cepa)* with curative powers. Hippocrates prescribed onions as diuretics, wound healers, and pneumonia fighters. In the Far East onions were used to treat infections. General Ulysses Grant believed onions were good for dysentery. And today, in the U.S. we believe onions are a healing food.

Onions Are Historically Healthy

There are more than 500 varieties of onions produced commercially around the globe. Most likely, the onion originally came from central Asia. And they have made their mark in history more than you'd ever imagine.

Ancient Greeks and Romans ate onions. Antony and Cleopatra (who had vinegar smarts) worshipped onions. They believed onions were a symbol of eternity. Why? Because of the circles that make up their structure.

Grecian athletes praised onions, too. Herodotus advised the first Olympic athletes to eat onions to "lighten the balance of the blood." To firm up their muscles, Gladiators were rubbed with onion juice.

In the Middle Ages, doctors prescribed onions as a remedy for headaches, snakebites, and hair loss.

(*Source:* National Onion Association.)

Like garlic, onions—"the rose among roots," according to Robert Louis Stevenson—are part of the healthful alluim family of vegetables. Research shows that medical benefits from eating onions regularly include reduced risk of cancer, heart disease, diabetes, and even asthma. And you can give credit to its nutrients.

According to the National Onion Association, there are few other vegetables that provide such high flavor and low calorie content. Onions combined with garlic, olive oil, and vinegar make a food recipe complete.

And garlic and onions are Mother Nature's healing combination. Research by Chinese scientists and the National Cancer Institute shows that eating more garlic and other bulb foods can lower the risk of getting stomach cancer. And that's not all.

Not only are onions healing with garlic, they are healthy solo, too. Good-for-you onions are low in sodium, contain several B vitamins, and like apple cider and red wine vinegar, are a good source of potassium—an important mineral for total good health.

Nutrition per Serving of Onions

Nutrient Composition

Serving Size: 1 large (150 grams, about 5.3 ounces)
Calories: 60
Protein (g): 174
Carbohydrates (g): 12.95
Total Lipid (Fat) (g): 0.24
Cholesterol: 0.0*
Sodium (mg): 4.5
Potassium (mg): 235.5
Vitamin A (mcg): 0.0

Vitamin C (mg): 9.6
Thiamin B_1 (mg): 0.06
Riboflavin B_2 (mg): 0.03
Niacin (mg): 0.22
Vitamin B_6 (mg): 0.17
Folate (mcg): 28.5
Calcium (mg): 30.0
Iron (mg): 0.33
Phosphorus (mg): 49.5
Magnesium (mg): 15.0
Copper (mg): 0.09
Dietary Fiber (g): 2.7

*Information on cholesterol content is provided for individuals who, on the advice of a physician, are modifying their total intake of cholesterol.

(*Source:* National Onion Association; Information provided by the USDA.)

Onions vs. Cancer. According to the NOA, quercetin, a powerful antioxidant, is also present in onions. Quercetin neutralizes free radicals in the body, and protects the membranes of the body's cells from damage. Preliminary research shows that quercetin may work to prevent cancer cells and blood clots from forming, adds the NAO.

In addition, the National Cancer Institute believes that a variety of chemicals in onions appear to inhibit the growth of cancer cells, especially of the gastrointestinal system, which means it can help prevent stomach cancer. Plus, according to reports, people in China's Shandong province, who eat large amounts of garlic and onions, cut their risk of stomach cancer as much as 40 percent.

Onions also can play a role in the five-a-day program, supported by the NCI, which is designed to help boost our intake of fruits and vegetables to at least five servings each day.

Here's how onions do their part, according to the NOA:

- Eat five servings of fruits and vegetables a day. (5½ ounces, uncooked, is considered one serving of onions.)
- Eat at least one vitamin A–rich selection each day. (Onions en-

hance other vegetables such as carrots, spinach, beets, or winter squash.)

- Eat at least one vitamin C–rich selection each day. (Onions are a source of vitamin C.)
- Eat at least one high-fiber selection each day. (Onions provide 2.7 grams of dietary fiber per serving.)
- Eat vegetables from the cabbage family several times a week. (Combine onions with cabbage in cooking or in salads and coleslaw.)

Onions vs. Heart Disease: Quercetin also seems to prevent blood clots from forming, which means onions can lower our risk of a stroke. Also, according to the NOA, onions have blood-thinning abilities because they contain another natural chemical, adenosine, which has been shown to lower blood levels of LDL or "bad" cholesterol in the blood. Plus, many heart patients are now advised to eat raw onions because they help increase blood circulation and reduce blood pressure and clotting.

Onions vs. Allergies: Red and yellow onions may boost your immunity to the allergic response. It's the anti-inflammatory compound quercetin—it acts a lot like the antihistamine cromolyn, that helps lessen allergies and asthma attacks.

OLIVE OIL AND VINEGAR

The olive tree was first cultivated in the Mediterranean countries 6,000 years ago. Since then, olive oil has played a therapeutic role in the diet and provides amazing healing powers, especially when combined with vinegar.

Olive oil is beneficial for the digestive system, brain power, and bone mineralization. It also protects against gallstones and stomach ulcers and helps relieve minor constipation, lower cholesterol levels, and guard against cancer, according to research by the International Olive Oil Council (IOOC).

Olive Oil and Your Health

Protection for	What It Does
Liver and gall bladder	Helps to produce evacuation of the gall bladder toward the intestine.
Intestines	Helps intestinal ingestion of fatty foods; oleical acid changes the fats' makeup so that they are assimilated in the intestine.
Arteries	Antioxidant vitamin E in olive oil fights free radicals and reduces the buildup of platelets, which helps prevent arteriosclerosis.
Skeleton	Oleical acid is vital for composition and growth in human bones.
Brain	Vitamin E, linolenic acid, and alpha-linolenic acid protect the brain from aging.

(*Source:* Brochure produced by Maison de l'Huile d' olive [Dr. Andre Charbonnier].)

Olive Oil vs. Heart Disease: Because of its biological effects, olive oil is the preferred fat by health experts for its cardiovascular benefits. Olive oil, which is 74 percent monounsaturated fat, is believed to increase the good cholesterol HDL, and lower the bad cholesterol LDL.

Olive Oil vs. Cancer: Olive oil, especially when included in the Mediterranean diet of vegetables, omega-3–rich fish, and fresh fruit, has been shown to help lower the risk of breast cancer.

While olive oil can help stave off heart disease and cancer, it seems to have antiaging effects as well. A few years ago, I did research for a *Woman's World* article on actress Loni Anderson's diet and how it keeps her young.

For one, the actor eats her greens. "I love a big leafy salad with olive oil," says Loni. Certain green vegetables, including Loni's favorites—broccoli, asparagus, and spinach—are full of antioxidant vitamins that may reduce wrinkles caused by repeated exposure to ultraviolet light, says Tufts University's Jeffrey Blumberg, Ph.D.

"I also throw garlic into practically everything,." Garlic is rich in the mineral selenium, an antioxidant that can help stall the aging process.

Good Fat versus Bad Fat

Saturated Fats	Monounsaturated Fats
• Fats from meats and poultry	• Peanut oil
• Palm kernel oil	• Olive oil
• Coconut oil	• Canola oil
• Fats from dairy products	

Types of Olive Oil

- *Extra virgin:* Extracted from the highest-quality olives. It must have less than 1 percent natural acidity. It's "fruity" flavor is intense and great in salads.
- *Virgin:* Processed mechanically (pressure) and without heat, which changes the oil's acidity to 1 to 5 percent. It's recommend for use in salad dressings and marinades.
- *Pure:* A mix of refined olive oil (treated with steam and chemicals) and virgin oils and is less costly. Acidity ranges from 3 to 4 percent. It's most often used in cooking.
- *Extracted and refined:* Made from whole cull olives and extracted during a second pressing with a chemical solvent; virgin oil is added for flavor.
- *Pomace:* Made by a chemical extraction of the residue leftover after crushing and second pressing of the olives. It contains 5 to 10 percent acidity; virgin oil is added for flavor.

I prefer to use extra virgin olive oil because it is the "crême" of the crop, so to speak. It makes my tossed green salads extra-special.

MEDITERRANEAN DIET

Garlic, onions, and olive oil—Mediterranean cuisine staples—are part of traditional and contemporary menus. We know Mediterraneans' diet includes these healthful ingredients which are key to helping reduce the risk of heart disease and cancer. And combined with red wine vinegar, their dishes are even healthier.

"Pastas, risottos, focaccias (Italian flat pizza bread), hefty salads—all those favorites at the local Italian restaurant—are just what the doctor ordered for good health and longevity. When travelers return from the Mediterranean crazy about the local food, they have fallen in love with Mother's Nature's own medicine," reports Nancy G. Freeman in her article on the Mediterranean Diet.[5]

Ah, the Mediterranean Diet. I can relate. For the past ten years I have practiced the traditional healthy Mediterranean Diet without knowing it. I eat plenty of breads, pasta, fruits, vegetables, olive oil, yogurt, fish, and poultry. And I eat very little sweets and red meat. At 46, I am a healthy, disease-free woman. It's got to be my diet.

Just chew on these Pro-Mediterranean facts[6]:

- Women of Greece have the lowest rate of breast cancer in the world.
- People living in countries that border the Mediterranean Sea have less cancer and heart disease than people in northern Europe and the United States.
- Mediterraneans live longer lives than northern Europeans and Americans.

Did you know that studies initiated by nutritionist Ancel Keys in the 1950s coined it the Mediterranean Diet? Its typical food stuffs include carbohydrates, fresh vegetables, fruits, salads, soups, fish, small amounts of red meat, and wine with meals.[7]

Also, Mediterraneans nix processed foods, forgo butter, and opt for olive oil, which accompanies salads, veggies, and is even used as a dip for focaccia. Keep in mind, however, it's not just what they eat—it's how they do it.[8]

Remember how it was in the fifties in America? We'd have regular, sit-down, *Leave It to Beaver* and *Ozzie and Harriet* meals. Three times a day. It was a time to eat and share with family and relatives. Well, now in 2000 we are a fast-paced society and eat on the run—kids and adults. But Mediterraneans do as we did. And it apparently has good health effects.

The Mediterranean diet—rich in vegetables, fruits, grains, beans, and fish—has once again been proven to be heart-protective. Researchers report that participants in the Lyon Diet Heart Study who had previously suffered heart attacks and who switched to the omega-3 fatty acid–rich diet had 47 to 72 percent lower risk of suffering a second heart attack or stroke.[9]

We know that fruits, vegetables, and whole grains—the crux of the Mediterranean diet—are brimming full of cancer-fighting antioxidants A, C, E, and other healthful compounds, too.

In fact, according to the American Cancer Society, vegetables and fruits are complex foods containing more than 100 beneficial vitamins, minerals, fiber, and other substances. And it's specific vitamins, minerals, fiber, and phytochemicals (again, those chemical compounds created by plants, such as carotenoids, flavonoids, termpenes, sterols, indoles, and phenols) that may help lower cancer risk.

Grains—which are part of the Mediterranean Diet—contain folate, calcium, and selenium, which are linked with a lower risk of colon cancer. And beans or legumes, another food Mediterraneans eat, are rich in vitamins, minerals, protein, and fiber, which may help guard against cancer and are a healthier high-protein option to meat.

Research is still in the works. Until we know exactly how each fruit and vegetable provides protection against cancer, the ACS recommends we eat five or more servings of fruits and vegetables a day, and six to eleven servings of grains.

Vinaigrette, Madam?

What do you get when you combine olive oil, wine vinegar, mustard, and a dash of ground pepper? Vinaigrette. The French will tell you that vinaigrette is the traditional salad dressing.

Today, this dressing is very popular because it's easy to make, tasty, and health-enhancing, too. While monounsaturated olive oil can help to keep your cholesterol levels in check, the vinegar adds a punch to your taste buds and will stave off a craving for salt.

The Traditional Healthy Mediterranean Diet Pyramid

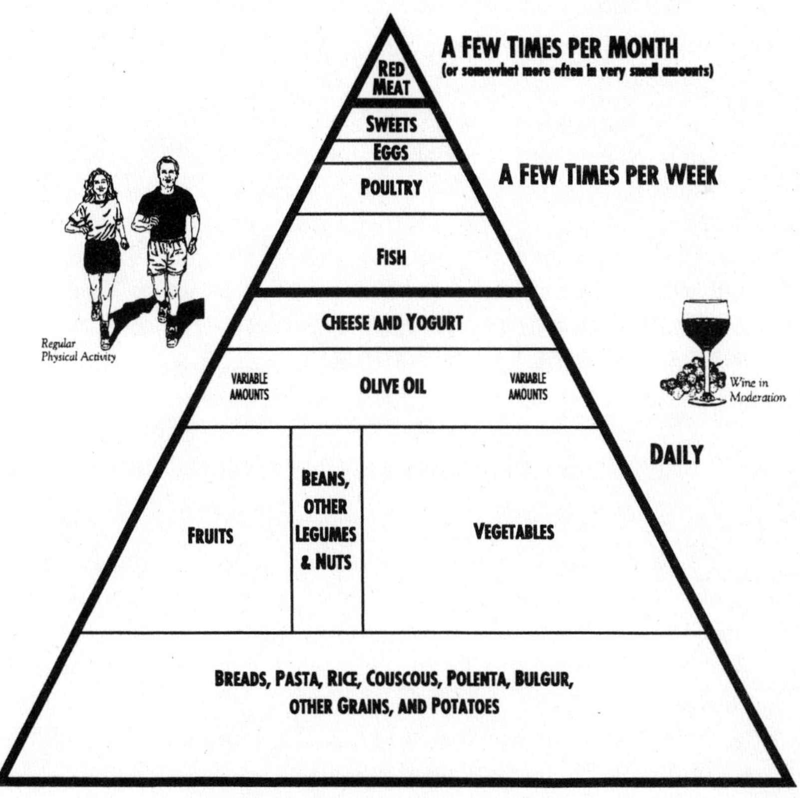

Vinaigrette Tips for You and Yours

Basic Vinaigrette: Mix ½ cup olive oil, 3–4 tablespoons red wine vinegar, ½ teaspoon Dijon mustard, and a dash of freshly ground pepper. Stir before putting on salad greens.

Storing Vinaigrette: A basic vinaigrette will stay fresh for up to 2 weeks in a sealed container in the refrigerator.

Storage Tips for Garlic, Onions, and Olive Oil

Garlic: Keep garlic in a cool, dry place with good circulation—not the refrigerator. Fresh garlic may keep for months. A bonus tip: Easy peeling? Plop a whole garlic clove in boiling water for about 5 seconds.

Onions: Keep onions, whole ones, in a cool, dry place with good ventilation—not the refrigerator. Wrap scallions and cut onions tightly in plastic wrap and refrigerate.

Olive Oil: You can store extra virgin olive oil up to 1 year after opening. Store it in a cool, dark place. Do not refrigerate it, but keep it away from heat.

Important Healing Hints to Remember

✓ Garlic's cholesterol-fighting organosulfur compounds can help keep heart disease at bay; may reduce risk of stomach cancer.

✓ Onions are heart-healthy due to the organosulfur compounds; and onions can help stave off stomach cancer because of their antioxidant quercetin. Onions may even help relieve asthma attacks.

✓ Olive oil contains squalene and has a high monounsaturated fat content—both are good for the heart.

✓ The Mediterranean Diet, which combines garlic, onions, and olive oil, is a healthful, heart-smart, anticancer way to eat.

CHAPTER

14

Vinegarmania: Hope or Hype?

A poet that fails in writing becomes often a morose critic; the weak and insipid white wine makes at length an excellent vinegar.

—William Shenstone

There's no doubt about it. Vinegar is hot these days. Not only can you find vinegar on the market and online, a variety of vinegar types are growing by leaps and bounds. What's more, while doctors use it, and plenty of people, like you and me, use it, even conventional associations are jumping on the vinegar wagon.

Sweet Vinegar Fact

Almost Everybody Does Vinegar: Who in the nation buys vinegar—and why? Ninety percent of American households use vinegar, although folks in the Pacific and Midatlantic states buy the most vinegar. Why? It may be due to the interest in salad and gourmet cooking in metropolitan areas. Also, during the late summer, vinegar sales soar because people buy gallons of vinegar for pickling and food preservation. The most popular food uses of vinegar are for salads, as a cooking ingredient, and for pickling and home canning.

(*Source:* Heinz U.S.A.)

The American Dietetic Association (ADA) encouraged consumers to load up your pantry with a "variety of vinegars." The association released the slogan for 1999 National Nutrition Month: "Take a fresh look at nutrition." The ADA suggests flavoring foods with things other than salt and fat. That means filling up your pantry with quick-fix items, including rice, pasta, beans, and a variety of vinegars, herbs, and other flavorings. And there's more.

VINEGAR STATISTICS

Supermarket Sales of All Types of Bottled Vinegar in Millions of Dollars

1998 $198.26
1997 $201.62
1996 $200.02
1995 $193.88
1994 $185.88
1993 $171.38

(*Source:* The Vinegar Institute; July 1999 issue of *Progressive Grocer Magazine* [part of Bill Communications in New York], which tracks sales of supermarkets having sales of $2 million or more. *Progressive Grocer* revised base dollar sales volumes in 1999, but the percent changes were not affected.)

Vinegar Retail Sale by Flavor

- 38% white distilled
- 21% cider
- 15% red wine
- 15% balsamic
- 6% rice
- 5% all other

(*Source:* Information Resources, Inc., 1997.)

Although bottled vinegar sold at retail makes up a large part of the vinegar market, vinegar is also a key ingredient in a number of familiar products. Vinegar adds flavor and zip to salad dressings, sauces, marinades, ketchup, mustard, pickles, tomato products, and more. Next time you're at the store, check out the ingredient statement on some of your favorite products—chances are vinegar makes the list.

Vinegar Distribution by Category, Percent

Bottled	33.7
Dressings and sauces	16.8
Pickles	14.8
Mustard	11.5
Other processed foods	10.5
Tomato products	8.5
Other	4.2

(*Source:* Vinegar Institute Production Survey, 1989.)

1997 Vinegar Purchasing Behavior

- In 1997, 52 percent of U.S. households purchased vinegar at least once.
- Each household spent about $3.57 per year on vinegar.
- Over 10 percent of the vinegar purchases involved some consumer-perceived deal (e.g., coupons, displays).

Q. ***Where do consumers buy vinegar?***
A. As the supermarket industry consolidates, other retail outlets such as mass merchandisers and drugstores are taking the opportunity to draw in consumers. The tables below provide insight into where and how much vinegar is purchase in various retail outlets.

(*Source:* The Vinegar Institute.)

Where Do Consumers Buy Vinegar?

Outlet	% buyers making at least one vinegar purchase in the retail outlet
Grocery store	91.8
Supermarket ($2 million+ sales)	89.6
Mass merchandiser	7.5
Supercenter	5.0
Warehouse club	4.8
Drug store	1.2
Convenience store	0.5

(*Source:* The Vinegar Institute; *Supermarket Business,* March 1999.)

1998 Vinegar Sales—Multichannel

Outlet	Dollar Sales (millions)	% Total Dollar Sales	% Change from
Supermarkets	$215.61	95.4	-2.2
Mass Merchandisers	9.27	4.1	19.1
Drugstores	1.13	0.5	18.7
3-Outlet Total	$226.01		

(*Source:* The Vinegar Institute; *Progressive Grocers,* July 1999, "1999 Sales Manual/Multichannel.")

Detoxify Your World

I remember as a little girl, my mother used white distilled vinegar to wash the windows inside and outside of our pink and white house in the suburbs. In my twenties, as a Denny's waitress, I remember using vinegar to wash out the coffeepots at the restaurant. In my thirties, as a college student, I used vinegar in the kitchen drain to get rid of odors. And today, I use vinegar for all those reasons—and more. Why?

We live in a very toxic world. And what better natural remedy to use for household purposes than natural vinegar? Science shows that many chemicals previously thought safe are not. The fact is, low levels of some common chemicals found in cleaning products can affect your immune and nervous systems.

I know firsthand how the body can be adversely affected by household chemicals. When I was in graduate school at San Francisco State University, I cleaned homes to pay for my tuition and living expenses. Three times a week (sometimes more) I'd clean houses for affluent people in Hillsborough and Palo Alto.

At first, even though I have always been a believer in natural foods, I didn't think twice about using harsh cleaning products. The oily furniture polish and strong-smelling shower cleaner got the job done.

As time passed, however, I began to experience some ill effects of those oh-so-powerful cleaning agents I valued. One time as I began to spray the shower, my employer grabbed her baby and dog and dashed for another room. I began to wonder, "If this cleaner is so toxic for infants and pets—what about me and my health?"

After a few bouts of coping with a runny nose or a sore throat, I wised up. I took a self-taught crash course on basic household cleaners. I began to read the labels of household cleaners (just like I read labels on food items). It was a wake-up call. But did you know that some chemical compounds in cleaning agents aren't even listed on the label?

The fact remains, there are toxic chemical compounds that are not safe for humans or animals. Here's some of the culprits:

ARE YOUR HOUSEHOLD CLEANERS MAKING YOU SICK?

Cleaning Chemical	Found in	Potential Side Effects
Ammonia	Glass cleaners, floor cleaners, furniture polishes	Irritates your eyes, nose, lungs; causes rashes, redness.
Bleach, mixed	Disinfectants, laundry bleaches, toilet bowl cleaner	Irritates the skin; when mixed with ammonia forms a toxic gas.

Formaldehyde	Disinfectants, furniture polishes, detergents	Nasal stuffiness, itchy red eyes, nausea, headache.
Glycols	Degreasers, dry-cleaning chemicals, floor cleaners	Irritates skin, eyes, nose, throat.
Lye	Tub and tile cleaners	Mixed with acids, lye can cause harmful vapors; splashed in eyes can cause blindness.
Napthalene	Air fresheners, carpet cleaners	Dangerous to breathe and can cause headaches nausea, confusion.
Petroleum distillates	Oven cleaners, pesticides	Irritate the skin.

The good news is, I switched to the natural stuff. One by one, I spoke to my clientele. Many of the women (especially the teacher with allergies; the multicat household owner; and housewife with multiple chemical sensitivity) did not mind that I insisted on using the natural household cleaners. In fact, we would make a nonchemical household cleaner list together. And white and cider vinegars were on the grocery list.

Here are some things you can do by using the "Kitchen Magician" to detoxify *your* household and planet.

DETOX YOUR KITCHEN

- **Disposal Fresh as a Rose.** To help keep your garbage disposal clean and fresh-smelling, try vinegar cubes. Mix one cup of vinegar in a sufficient amount of water to fill an ice tray. Freeze the mixture and run the cubes through the disposal. After the grinding action has stopped, flush with cold water for a minute or so.
- **Dishwasher Fresh.** To help keep the drain line on your dishwasher clean and fresh-smelling, add one-half cup of white vinegar to the rinse cycle.
- **Fixtures That Sparkle Bright.** Remove soap and stain buildup on

chrome and plastic fixtures by cleaning with a mixture of 1 teaspoon salt dissolved in 2 tablespoons of white vinegar.

- **Shine on Counters.** Clean formica tabletops and counters by rubbing with a cloth soaked in white vinegar. The finish will shine. (Trust me on this one.)
- **Stamp Out Grease.** Dampen your cleaning rag in vinegar and water and use it to wipe out your oven. It will prevent grease buildup.
- **Mr. Dishwashing Magic.** To remove chalky deposits left on dinnerware and glasses, place affected pieces in dishwasher. Place cup filled with vinegar on bottom rack. Run the machine for 5 minutes. Stop the machine and empty cup which is now filled with water. Refill with vinegar and complete cycle. Follow by a complete cycle with dishwasher detergent.

Personal Protection

- **Put Out Smoky Odors.** To remove smoky odors from clothes, fill a bathtub with hot water and add 1 cup of white vinegar. Hang the garments above the steaming bath water.
- **Freshen Up Baby!** Baby's clothes will be fresher if you add 1 cup of white vinegar to each load during the rinse cycle. Vinegar naturally breaks down uric acid and soapy residue in diapers, leaving the clothes soft and fresh.
- **Easy Wash Silks.** To wash silks at home, add a half capful of Woolite® and 2 tablespoons of white vinegar to 2 quarts of very cold water. Dunk clothes up and down in the mixture but do not soak. Dry just enough to iron by rolling in a Turkish towel and pressing while still damp. You may wish to test a particular item by dipping the tail of the blouse or detachable tie before doing the entire piece.
- **Sock It to the Suds.** Get rid of excess suds that billow up during hand laundry by adding a splash of vinegar to the second rinse. Then rinse again in plain water.
- **Gentle Hand Helper.** To restore moisture to hands when they have been in strong cleaning solutions, plaster, concrete, or powdered detergents, simply rub them with vinegar.
- **Cola Spots Fizzle.** To remove cola-based soft drink spots from

100% cotton, polyester and cotton blends, and permanent press cotton fabrics, sponge the stain within 24 hours. Apply undiluted vinegar directly to the stain and rub away the marks. Launder or dry clean according to the manufacturer's care tag instructions.

- **Goodbye Wine Stains.** To remove wine stains from 100% cotton, polyester and cotton blends, and permanent press fabrics, sponge the stain with full strength vinegar. Treat the stain within 24 hours and wash and dry as directed on the manufacturer's care tag instructions.
- **No More Catsup.** For catsup stains in 100% cotton, permanent press, and polyester cotton materials, sponge stain with undiluted vinegar within 24 hours. Wash immediately.
- **Lime Fighter.** Lawn and garden lime washes off the hands readily with a dousing of vinegar. Follow with a cold water rinse and apply skin lotion if desired.

NONTOXIC FLOOR CLEANERS

- **No-Wax Linoleum.** To wash no-wax linoleum, add one-half cup of white vinegar to a half-gallon of warm water. Your floor will become sparkling clean.
- **Liven Up Carpet.** To bring up the color in rugs and carpets, brush them with a mixture of 1 cup of white vinegar to a gallon of water.

NATURAL BATHROOM CLEANUP

- **Good Riddance Bathtub Film.** To remove film buildup on bathtubs, wipe with vinegar and then soda. Rinse clean with water.
- **Natural Bowl Cleaner.** Got kids and pets so you're nervous about using bleach in the bowl? Clean it the natural way. Pour undiluted white vinegar into it. Let it stand for 5 minutes and then flush. Stubborn stains may be removed by spraying them with vinegar and brushing vigorously. (Works like a charm, really!)
- **Unclog Showerhead.** To remove corrosion from showerhead or faucet, soak them in diluted white vinegar overnight. For convenience, saturate a cloth in vinegar and wrap it around the faucet or showerhead.

- **Shower Curtain Clean.** Nothing is better than a brand-new shower curtain. After a while, though, it begins to look spotty with soap film. Toss your favorite plastic shower curtains in the washing machine with a bath towel. During the rinse cycle, add 1 cup of white vinegar. Then, tumble dry briefly. (I've put this on my To Do list.)

Miscellaneous Nontoxic Household Uses

- **Lose the Ants.** Ants are pesky. And using toxic chemicals to zap them is worse. Opt to wash countertops, cabinets, and floors with equal parts of vinegar and water to deter ant invasions the natural way. (Good idea. I don't want my senior Fido and Fluffy exposed to toxins.)
- **Chrome Polish Perfect.** To polish chrome and stainless steel, simply moisten a cloth with white vinegar and wipe clean.
- **Wood Paneling Delight.** Wood paneling is beautiful. To keep it looking good, mix 1 ounce of olive oil with 2 ounces of white vinegar and 1 quart of warm water. Dampen a soft cloth with the solution and wipe the paneling. Then wipe with a dry, soft cloth to remove yellowing from surface.
- **Meltdown Dust.** Got a stubborn ring resulting from wet glasses being placed on wood furniture (water or alcohol)? Don't despair. Rub with a mixture of equal parts olive oil and white vinegar. A bonus tip: Rub with the grain, then polish.
- **Fresh as a Daisy.** Everyone wants to keep fresh-cut flowers fresh longer. Just add 2 tablespoons of vinegar plus 3 tablespoons of sugar to each quart of warm water (100° F). Keep flower stems in 3–4 inches of water to allow constant flow of nourishment.
- **Rx for Wobbly Furniture.** Ready to toss out old chairs or tables? Instead apply vinegar with a small oil can. It will loosen old glue around rungs and joints.

Keep It Green Outside

- **Bye Bye Grass.** To kill grass on sidewalks and driveways, pour full-strength vinegar on it.

- **Fuel Forever.** To make gasoline or propane lantern mantles last longer, soak them for several hours in vinegar and allow them to dry before using. They'll burn brighter on the same amount of fuel.
- **Cut That Rust.** To free a rusted or corroded bolt, soak it in vinegar.

(*Source:* The Vinegar Institute.)

LIGHTEN UP WITH VINEGAR FENG SHUI

You may have heard about Feng Shui, an age-old practice that holds the idea of living in harmony and balance with our environment. Now think of Martha Stewart and her beautiful household tips. Then, think vinegar. That's right, vinegar. Infused vinegar, that is.

Feng Shui is often used in homes, and can be very valuable when you place special objects in a room. Now take those flavored vinegars you made and line them along a windowsill to catch the sunlight. It will show off their healthful ingredients—parsley, sage, rosemary, and other herbs.

And remember, at the same time the seasonings infuse their flavor into vinegar and olive oil, to be used later for tasty recipes. Taking that special bottle (or two) of infused vinegar out of the shelf and placing it along a windowsill can make your living environment healthier and you may feel more connected to the life forces which surround us.

Show Your Stuff

- Flavored vinegars look great on kitchen countertops.
- Be creative when selecting containers.
- Choose ceramic or glass bottles with secure lids.
- Display herb vinegar in clear glass.
- Find elegantly detailed bottles at flea markets, garage sales, or antique stores, or order them from specialty catalogs or cookery stores.
- Prevent vinegar from clouding by sterilizing your containers first.

(*Source:* Heinz U.S.A.)

VINEGAR BEAUTIFUL

The following healthful vinegar beauty recipes are all natural and without harsh toxic chemicals:

- **Recipe 1: Vinegar to Aid Oily Skin.** One pint apple cider vinegar, 1 cup each lavender petals, lemon rind, rose petals, and sage. Steep this in a sunny window in a dark, glass jar that's well sealed for 3 weeks. Shake daily, then strain and rebottle.
- **Recipe 2: Vinegar for Dry Skin.** The same as the first recipe but use chamomile, mint, parsley, and primrose petals instead.
- **Recipe 3: Astringent/Hair Rinse.** Use white wine vinegar to which you add 1 cup orange peel (and if possible a half-cup orange leaves). Follow same procedure.
- **Recipe 4: Alternative Astringent for Your Skin.** Use any type of vinegar to which 1 cup of chopped marigolds has been added. This will dry pimples and also help heal minor scrapes.

(*Source:* Patricia Telesco, Amherst, New York.)

Martha Washington's Famous Facial

In 1754, during the French and Indian War, Martha Custis bewitched George Washington at a dance. The legend is, that from across the dance floor it was her radiant complexion that caught his eye—and won his heart. The two married four years later. So what was Martha's beauty secret that made a big statement? Vinegar, ladies. Here's the famous facial mask:

Beat 1 egg, separate, till frothy. Combine the egg, 1 teaspoon honey, and ¼ teaspoon apple cider vinegar. Apply to your face and neck. After 15–20 minutes, rinse with warm water and dry.[1]

Important Healing Hints to Remember

- ✓ Vinegar statistics prove that vinegar is more popular today than ever.
- ✓ Vinegar can clean and detox your entire house, naturally.
- ✓ By placing beautiful infused vinegar bottles in your household space, you can healthy up your mind and spirit.
- ✓ Natural vinegar can help beautify your hair and skin.
- ✓ The healing powers of vinegar may not be for everyone.

PART 6

VINEGAR REMEDIES

CHAPTER

15

Therapeutic Uses

Nature opened the first drugstore.[1]
—D. C. Jarvis, M.D.

Chances are, apple cider, red wine, rice, and other vinegars—your everyday household products—contain even *more* extraordinary healing powers that you might not know about. The next time you need a natural remedy for a minor ailment, check this list first to see if a cure is as close as your kitchen cabinet or pantry.

I'll describe thirty common health ailments and cosmetic uses, from A to Z, and provide common at-home vinegar folk remedies. Some treatments can be used inside and others outside the body. Keep in mind, these are based on anecdotal evidence. There are no clinical double-blind studies to back up their effectiveness and make it conclusive. But first, just listen to real stories from real people, like you and me, who have medical uses for vinegar and vow that it can and really does work!

"It Worked for Me!" Real Stories About Vinegar

Personal stories often are even more convincing than statistics, studies, and even doctors' advice. Here, take a look at real-life people. You be the judge.

Bee Stings

I have a high regard for vinegar since it has come to my rescue more than once. I was stung on the hand by a bee while in the garden one day. The sting was very painful and frightening. I came running into the house, yelling to my husband that I'd been stung. I proceeded to tell him how painful it was.

I'm the nurse in the family so I should have known what to do, but sometimes when the injury is to yourself and you're in a lot of pain, you don't. My dear husband took over; he told me all about the vinegar book he was reading and how vinegar would take the pain away. I was quite leery. I knew that vinegar was acetic acid and I was afraid it would make it hurt more. My husband poured vinegar over my inflamed finger and within 15 seconds the pain was completely gone! The finger never swelled and the redness that had already started went away completely! I had no more pain and I was able to go on with my day and use my hand like nothing had ever happened![2]

—Bonnie K. McMillen, R.N.

Plantar Warts

The next time vinegar came to my rescue was for an ongoing problem I was having with plantar warts on the bottom of my foot. I contracted the pesky virus from the local Y's locker room floor. It was spreading and I was dreading going to the podiatrist because I knew it would involve money and pain. Instead, I luckily thought of vinegar . . . it had saved me before . . . could it get rid of plantar warts? I decided it was worth a try. I soaked my foot about three times a week. I should have done it every night but I just couldn't remember to do it every night. Nothing happened for about 2–3 weeks but I was determined to make life on my foot very uncomfortable for these warts. So after every soak I would rub my foot vigorously with a clean towel. Finally after about 2–3 weeks I noticed the nasty little black warts were loosening their grip on my foot and some were being toweled away!

This was incredible but it made perfect sense! Salicylic acid is the common ingredient in over-the-counter remedies for treating warts, and vinegar is acetic acid . . . still an acid but a much gentler treatment. I continued to soak my foot every night and within 5–6 weeks or so from the beginning of treatment the 15 or 20 warts were completely gone and have not recurred. I also learned to wear shower shoes at the gym and to never walk around a locker room or pool area in my bare feet.[3]

—Bonnie K. McMillen, R.N.

Sunburn

I remember getting the worst sunburn of my life on a Florida beach. I did not use sunscreen, but at the time I was taking Bactrim, and completely forgot about the warnings to avoid the sun while taking that medication. The result was a sunburn so painful and blistering that I could not even sit down comfortably. I took some acetaminophen and whined a lot. Then our neighbor suggested using white vinegar on the sunburn. I will never forget the relief that the vinegar provided.[4]

—Carol Mulvihill

Burns

In the spring of 1956, I was 18 years old and living in Sacramento with my parents. One evening after frying bacon, I was draining off the boiling grease when the handle on the frying pan broke and the grease spilled all over my right palm and fingers. Needless to say, it hurt a great deal. All the emergency room doctors could do was put some sort of cream on it and a bandage and suggest I immerse the hand in cold water to ease the pain. Big help that was! Took quite a while to heal.

Many years later, 1970 I think, while yet again frying bacon for my three sons and me, the handle on the frying pan broke loose and once again boiling grease flowed over my right palm and fingers. Oddly enough it was the same frying pan my father had put a new handle on, and up till then it worked fine. But this time I was prepared!

I had been delving into metaphysical healing, and of the many things I came across was using "apple cider vinegar" on burns. So I quickly and calmly poured the vinegar over my hand and intoned the prayer, "I am now perfectly healed in the name of Jesus Christ our Lord!" Immediately upon looking at both my palms, it was impossible to tell which one had been burned. The hand was perfect. To this day, we always use the vinegar and prayer for any burns of any kind, with the same healing results.

—Mrs. Janice Oszust

Thirty Amazing Vinegar Remedies

1 ZAP ACNE Acne plagues not only teenagers, but adult women too. More than 17 million American women—in their twenties, thirties, and forties—suffering from postadolescent outbreaks of adult acne. "Adult acne is characterized by the same type of pimples that mark the faces of youngsters," says Dr. William Epstein, professor of dermatology at the University of California, San Francisco.

If you have acne, genetics may be the primary cause. Unfortunately, some of us are born with acne-prone pores. Yet if you're predisposed to mild acne, you can keep it under control with vinegar.

What Vinegar Remedy to Use: To get rid of acne, make a mixture of 2 teaspoons of plain or herbal apple cider vinegar in 1 cup of water and dab on blemishes several times a day after washing.

Why You'll Like It: If you already have acne, you know the physical pain and self-consciousness it can create. Instead of having to go out and buy acne medicine, you can go to your kitchen cabinet. Not only is ACV readily available but it costs pennies to use. The best part is, it can help dry up blemishes.

2 TAME ARTHRITIS Folk medicine holds that ACV can help fight arthritis. While no scientific studies prove this to be true, and conventional doctors frown at the thought of vinegar as an antiarthritis remedy, testimony gives nutrient-rich apple cider vinegar kudos for providing relief for the debilitating disease.

What Vinegar Remedy to Use: The popular remedy is simple. Take 2 spoonfuls of apple cider vinegar and honey in a glass of water several times daily.

Why You'll Like It: If it works for you, you will be happy because it's natural, which means there will be no ill side effects from pain medications. Plus, it's low-cost and easy to apply.

3 PERKY ASTRINGENT An astringent can help close facial pores and refresh the skin. An ancient formula created by the gypsies in the 5th century was used by the Queen of Hungary.

What Vinegar Remedy to Use: Mix red wine vinegar, witch hazel extract, pure rose water, rosemary, and rose fragrance.

Why You'll Like It: Not only can this help perk up your skin, it can be used as an after-bath, after-wash, or after-shave, too.

4 WALK OUT ON ATHLETE'S FOOT Athlete's foot is a form of fungus infection of the feet. The fact is, athlete's foot doesn't happen among people who go barefoot. It's moisture, sweating, and lack of proper air of the feet that provide the ideal setting for athlete's foot to grow.

What Vinegar Remedy to Use: Rinse your feet several times a day with plain or herbal apple cider vinegar. I can personally attest that it burns, then soothes the skin between the toes and redness.

Why You'll Like It: Apple cider vinegar may relieve the itching of athlete's foot. Better yet, it can help prevent it, too. It's acid content helps stop fungus growth. A bonus: Apple cider vinegar is not as messy as prescription ointments.

5 SOOTHE AND HEAL BURNS Ever burn yourself on the stovetop, iron, or fireplace? Ouch! Any burn that affects your body should be attended to ASAP. The reason: You'll want to keep inflammation and swelling at a minimum.

What Vinegar Remedy to Use: Apply apple cider vinegar, straight out of the bottle, to a burn on the surface of the body. Better still, apply ice cold vinegar right away for fast relief.

Why You'll Like It: It may help alleviate smarting and soreness and prevent blisters.

6 SMOOTH CHAPPED SKIN During the dry, cold winter months, dry skin can be a problem from head to toe. If you can't fly off to the Bahamas, what's the next best thing to do? Take a vinegar vacation.

What Vinegar Remedy to Use: Mix your best hand cream and vinegar. Apply this vinegar cream each time after you wash your hands.

Why You'll Like It: If your hand cream is made of natural ingredients, you will have a natural product that can soothe, smooth, and heal hands fast naturally.

7 CLEAR UP CONGESTION When it comes to fighting colds and sinus congestion, apple cider vinegar comes to the rescue, according to folk medicine.

What Vinegar Remedy to Use: To clear up clogged respiratory congestion, inhale a vapor mist from a steaming pot containing water and several spoonfuls of vinegar.

Why You'll Like It: It will help clear the air passages naturally, and you'll be breathing easy again.

8 TAKE OFF CORNS Corns are the most common condition of the foot. Simply put, a corn is a thickening of the outer layer of skin—often at the tops of the toes.

What Vinegar Remedy to Use: Combine two slices of white bread and two onion slices with 1 cup of vinegar for one day. Put the bread on your corn, top with a slice of onion, and wrap with a bandage overnight.

Why You'll Like It: It is a creative folk remedy that can be fun and worth the time and effort if it works.

9 DUMP DANDRUFF If you suffer from dry flakes and dry scalp, you are hardly alone. Skin complaints can be helped with external use of vinegar. It is thought that the vinegar kills the bacteria which is believed to be the cause.

What Vinegar Remedy to Use: Massage a small amount of apple cider vinegar directly into the washed scalp, leave on for up to 1 minute, then rinse. Repeat this regimen daily until the flakes are gone.

Why You'll Like It: Apple cider vinegar is a safe and nontoxic remedy, whereas many dandruff shampoos on the market are chock-full of toxic chemicals. Plus, vinegar costs much, much less.

10 DOUCHE SMART As a child of the fifties, I remember a pink douche bag hanging up on the towel rack in my mother's shower stall.

In my twenties, buying ready-to-use disposable douching products (scented) was the trendy thing to do. And I did it.

But that was the seventies. Things have changed. Today, some experts believe frequent douching may endanger a woman's health. It may increase a woman's risk of a vaginal infection and even her risk of cervical cancer.

But if you have chronic vaginal infections, medical doctors believe that an occasional douche can be helpful. What's more, if you have trichomonas (a one-celled organism causing a vaginal infection) while pregnant, rather than taking the prescribed Flagyl, a vinegar and water douche is recommended.

What Vinegar Remedy to Use: Dr. Mike Samuels of San Francisco suggests 2 tablespoons of white vinegar to a quart of water. "Vinegar changes the acid balance of the vagina to one which makes it more difficult for the monilia to grow," he says.

Why You'll Like It: For your health's sake, bear in mind that infrequent douching—once a week or less—with a mild solution of vinegar is safer than other strong chemical preparations.

11 FADE FRECKLES Although some people like the freckle look, many women want to lighten up freckles on the body.

What Vinegar Remedy to Use: Popular folk medicine believers claim that you can lighten freckles from neck to toe (not your face) by applying horseradish vinegar.

Why You'll Like It: Rather than use a harsh facial product to remove freckles, a natural remedy, like vinegar, may do the trick without ill side effects.

12 LOSE THE HEADACHE The most common type of headache is the tension headache. It feels like a rubber band is being tightened around your head. And let's face it, almost everyone has or will experience at least one whopper.

What Vinegar Remedy to Use: To get rid of a tension headache, dab an herbal vinegar on your temples and lie down. Or dampen a cloth with the vinegar and put it on your forehead.

For relieving migraines, Dr. Jarvis recommends a vinegar vapor. Mix equal parts of vinegar and water in a pan on the stove and bring it to a boil. Lean your head over the pan and inhale the fumes for 75 breaths.

Why You'll Like It: If you have ever endured a headache, you will appreciate any remedy that works. And if it's easily accessible, like vinegar, and without the side effects that aspirin can have, all the better.

13 STOP HICCUPS When the diaphragm gets irritated, it pushes up and makes your breath come out abnormally—and you let out a "Hic!" The causes can vary from eating too fast or too much to overexcitement.

What Vinegar Remedy to Use: Sip a glass of warm water with 1 teaspoon of vinegar mixed in it. I suggest drinking from the far side of a glass for antihiccup double effect.

Why You'll Like It: It beats having someone jump out and scare you, and has fewer calories than putting sugar in a glass of water.

14 STAVE OFF IMPETIGO This streptococcus infection of the skin is very, very contagious. I remember as a preteenager my girlfriend's best friend had impetigo on her chin. My mother was very wary and warned us to keep our hands to ourselves.

What Vinegar Remedy to Use: Apply apple cider vinegar straight from the bottle on each infected area of the skin.

Why You'll Like It: If the home remedy works, it prevents a doctor bill and will stop an impetigo epidemic in your neighborhood.

15 SWAT INSECT AND BEE STINGS Ouch! Bug bites hurt first, itch later. And nobody likes to look at red bump and lumps. Mosquitoes, bees, and ants, oh my! What's an outdoor and indoor human to do?

What Vinegar Remedy to Use: Make yourself more comfortable in a homemade paste made from vinegar and cornstarch. Apply it directly to the bumps and blisters.

Why You'll Like It: It soothes the itch and dries out blisters.

16 LOSE THE LAMENESS Walking s-l-o-w can occur for many reasons, from too much exercise or not enough. Whatever the cause, lameness can be painful. But there is a liniment that may provide relief.

What Vinegar Remedy to Use: In his book, Dr. Jarvis recommends to beat up the yolk of one egg with 1 tablespoon of turpentine and 1 tablespoon of apple cider vinegar. Rub into the skin.[5]

Why You'll Like It: If it relieves lameness, you'll like it.

17 GOOD RIDDANCE TO MORNING SICKNESS Nausea and vomiting often in the A.M. are common in almost half of all pregnant women. Morning sickness starts the first month of pregnancy and can last until the fourteenth to sixteenth week. The cause is unknown; however, it may be due to hormones or lower blood sugar during pregnancy.

What Vinegar Remedy to Use: To relieve morning sickness, as soon as you rise drink a glass of water with a teaspoon of apple cider vinegar.

Why You'll Like It: Morning sickness sufferers will gladly use any remedy that has a chance of beating the A.M. blahs.

18 Rx FOR MUSCLE CRAMPS Ever wake up in the middle of the night and cringe at that sharp, painful muscle cramp? They can strike the feet, legs, and even the stomach. What to do?

What Vinegar Remedy to Use: Doctors Patricia and Paul Bragg recommend taking 2 teaspoons apple cider vinegar and 1 teaspoon of honey in a glass of distilled water three times per day.

Why You'll Like It: It may work, claim the Braggs, by allowing the precipitated acid crystals in your circulatory system to enter into a solution and pass out of the body.

19 FIGHT OFF NIGHT SWEATS Ever have a bad case of the flu? Sometimes before it hits, in the middle of the night, you'll wake up in the wee A.M. hours and your sheets will be drenched. Eek! Also, menopausal women may experience night sweats in between hot flashes (not something to look forward to).

What Vinegar Remedy to Use: Try a sponge bath of apple cider vinegar at bedtime.

Why You'll Like It: This Vermont folk medicine remedy offers you help in preventing night sweats.

20 HERE'S TO GOOD PET HEALTH Even cats, dogs, and horses can benefit from vinegar. Holistic veterinarians such as Bob Goldstein, V.M.D., of Westport, Connecticut, believes organic apple cider vinegar is food for your pet's coat and for cleansing the body of toxins. "The natural acidity helps regulate digestion, and the pectin helps keep the intestines in good shape."[6]

What Vinegar Remedy to Use: Add 1 tablespoon apple cider vinegar to your cat or dog's water bowl.

Why You'll Like It: Anything natural that can enhance your pet's good health and longevity will make them wag their tail and you will wag yours, too.

21 ACV CAN PREVENT STONES IN HORSES Enteroliths, commonly known as stones, form in the large intestines of horses. Veterinarians at the University of California–Davis have seen many horses suffering from this health ailment. Removal of stones can cost more than $3,500 for surgery and postoperative care.

What Vinegar Remedy to Use: The good news is, diet can play a preventive role. According to Douglas L. Langer, D.V.M., oat or grass hay tends to be lower in minerals and doesn't seem to maintain the high pH linked with alfalfa hay. Grain—and even apple cider vinegar—can also be good since it promotes a lower intestinal pH. UC Davis vets recommend 1–2 cups per day as a preventive measure.

Why You'll Like It: Use caution, some horses do develop a loose stool from the feeding of vinegar. If this happens, discontinue, but after the stools are normal, find the right vinegar solution that does not produce loose stools for your horse.[7]

22 RUB OUT POISON IVY, OAK, AND SUMAC These three Canadian plants—poison ivy, western poison oak, and poison sumac—contain a poisonous sap that causes dermatitis—a pesky skin disorder.

Symptoms include severe itching of the skin and oozing sores. While most cases of poisoning go away in 7–10 days, you can find relief without going to the drugstore.

What Vinegar Remedy to Use: Neal Schultz, M.D., a dermatologist in New York, recommends two vinegar solutions: mix equal parts vinegar and rubbing alcohol and apply to rash. Be sure to wash—thoroughly—plus everything that came in contact with the plant. Or mix equal parts buttermilk, vinegar, and salt and apply.

Why You'll Like It: These homemade vinegar pastes have a chemical that draws out the poison—so it relieves the burning and itching of the skin like calamine lotion.

23 ROUND UP RINGWORM *Tinea corporis* is caused by your body's response to advancing fungi. Lesions appear in a circular shape—with a raised border. Worse, inflammation and itching sets in.

What Vinegar Remedy to Use: Dr. Jarvis recommends applying apple cider vinegar with your fingers to the ringworm area six times daily.

Why You'll Like It: Since apple cider vinegar is antiseptic, it may help treat ringworm.

24 STAMP OUT SHINGLES My neighbor had shingles. She sheepishly confessed to me how painful the skin area on her chest was where the shingles were located.

What Vinegar Remedy to Use: Dr. Jarvis recommends dabbing apple cider vinegar directly on the shingles. Repeat four times daily and three times during the night.

Why You'll Like It: You'll find instant relief of the itching and burning in the skin, and the shingles may heal faster.

25 BABY THAT SUNBURN Exposure to ultraviolet rays in sunlight is the primary cause of sunburn. Sunburns can cause short-term redness, pain, blistering, and fever. Long-term skin damage includes premature aging and skin cancer.

While we know sun exposure is unhealthy, sometimes a sunburn is inevitable. But vinegar comes to the rescue. Treatment includes applying cold compresses to the burned area.

What Vinegar Remedy to Use: Apply ice cold vinegar immediately for fast relief.

Why You'll Like It: It will prevent blisters. My mother put cold compresses of red wine vinegar and ice on my very red back and thighs after a bad burn at the beach. It did its job.

26 STOP SWIMMER'S EAR A common ailment that I remember getting as a teenage competitive swimmer. You can develop this ailment by swimming and showering as well.

What Vinegar Remedy to Use: To protect against ear infections from swimming pools, a popular folk remedy to try is using a mixture of one part white vinegar to one part rubbing alcohol.

Why You'll Like It: Vinegar is a good preventive strategy that can help keep pesky swimmer's ear at bay, while you splash in the pool or indulge in long showers.

27 ATTEND TO THAT TOOTHACHE While an aching tooth is a good sign that you need dental attention, sometimes temporary relief is necessary especially if the pain starts in the middle of the night or if you are out of town. That's where vinegar comes into play.

What Vinegar Remedy to Use: One popular remedy is to dab a cotton swab soaked in acacia vinegar.

Why You'll Like It: Like oil of cloves, this natural vinegar remedy may provide temporary relief. And you won't compound your misery with the ill side effects of pain medications.

28 SOOTHE A SORE THROAT When you feel the sniffles or flu coming on, a sore throat is often a symptom. While healing foods like vitamin C–rich citrus juices can lessen the severity of an illness, vinegar may help relieve that scratchy, painful feeling in your throat that makes it so hard to swallow.

What Vinegar Remedy to Use: To get rid of a painful sore throat, gargle with a 50–50 solution of warm water and vinegar.

Why You'll Like It: It is easy to do, all-natural, and doesn't have the sugar or chemicals that many sore throat lozenges contain.

29 GAIN WEIGHT While countless Americans struggle with obesity, there are a lot of people who want to put on the pounds. According to the Braggs, underweight people lack natural enzymes and food is not utilized by the body.

What Vinegar Remedy to Use: The good doctors suggest drinking 1 teaspoon apple cider vinegar and 1 teaspoon honey in a glass of distilled water upon rising. "Add to this 2 drops of liquid iodine made from seaweed, available in health stores. This adds natural iodine, which is so important to body health, and helps normalize body weight up or down as needed," they claim.

Why You'll Like It: Natural apple cider vinegar is healthier than loading up on high-fat fare. And it may be more palatable to you than caloric protein drinks and less costly!

30 ALOHA VARICOSE VEINS It's estimated that more than two-thirds of all American women and half of all men in the United States have swollen veins that appear near the surface of the skin. While they are unsightly, they can ache, too. Some natural remedies include: watch your weight, and avoid constipation. Perhaps that's why fiber-rich apple cider vinegar is the ticket to shrinking spider veins.

What Vinegar Remedy to Use: Dr. Jarvis reports that his patients taught him to apply apple cider vinegar straight to the varicose veins at morning and night. Plus, he recommends taking 2 teaspoons of vinegar in a glass of water twice a day.[8]

Why You'll Like It: Dr. Jarvis's patients got results, so mark your calendar. You, too, will notice shrinkage in 30 days.

Important Healing Hints to Remember

If it doesn't specify which type of vinegar to use, go ahead and use your own preference: an apple cider vinegar, a red wine vinegar, or a white vinegar.

Ailment	Vinegar	What It May Do
✓ Acne	Plain or herbal apple cider vinegar	Gets rid of blemishes
✓ Arthritis	Apple cider vinegar	Relieves soreness
✓ Astringent	Red wine vinegar	Perk up skin
✓ Athlete's foot	Plain or herbal apple cider vinegar	Soothes burning
✓ Skin burns	Apple cider vinegar	Lessen soreness
✓ Chapped skin	Vinegar	Heals
✓ Congestion	Apple cider vinegar	Reduces mucus
✓ Corns	Vinegar	Gets rid of corns
✓ Dandruff	Apple cider vinegar	Fights flakes
✓ Douche	White vinegar	Mild, safe
✓ Freckles	Horseradish vinegar	Fades spots
✓ Headache	Herbal vinegar	Provide headache relief
✓ Hiccups	Vinegar	Hiccups will stop
✓ Impetigo	Apple cider vinegar	Heals the skin
✓ Morning sickness	Apple cider vinegar	Subdues nausea
✓ Muscle cramps	Apple cider vinegar	It may excrete acid crystals
✓ Night sweats	Apple cider vinegar	Controls sweating
✓ Poison oak/ivy/sumac	Vinegar	Relieves itching/burning

Ailment	Vinegar	What It May Do
✓ Ringworm	Apple cider vinegar	Dries it up
✓ Shingles	Apple cider vinegar	Relieves burning/itching
✓ Sore throat	Vinegar	Relieves soreness
✓ Sunburn	Red wine vinegar	Relieves pain
✓ Toothache	Acacia vinegar	Relieves pain temporarily
✓ Varicose Veins	Apple cider vinegar	Shrinks the veins
✓ Weight gain	Apple cider vinegar	Helps metabolism

CHAPTER

16

Vinegar Is Not for Everyone: Some Sour Views

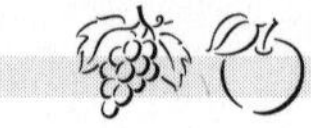

Of such vinegar aspect
That they'll not show their teeth by way of smile
Though Nestor swear the jest be laughable.
—William Shakespeare, *The Merchant of Venice*[1]

Versatile vinegar can be used inside and outside your body. But internal use of different vinegars may not be ideal for some people, according to Susan M. Lark, M.D., of Los Altos, California. In her latest book *Chemistry of Success*, she discusses the pH and alkaline mineral content of vinegar.

In Dr. Lark's clinical practice, she has found that consumption of certain acidic, low-pH foods such as different types of vinegar can be stressful to overly acidic people—despite vinegar's potential nutritional perks.

"The reason for this is that their highly acidic pH can trigger either immediate or slower-acting stress responses within the body," she reports. Also, adds Dr. Lark, many of her overly acidic patients have complained about vinegar causing unpleasant reactions such as canker sores, heartburn, bladder pain, and joint discomfort.[2]

"Other potentially nutritious but highly acidic foods like tomatoes, pineapple, raspberries, and wine can also cause similar symptoms. Repeated consumption of these low-pH foods tends to trigger chronic damage, inflammation, and overacidity in the affected tissues of sensitive people."[3]

The following chart provided by Dr. Lark compares the pH and alkaline mineral content (i.e. calcium, magnesium, potassium, and sodium) of various flavoring agents—including apple cider vinegar:

pH AND ALKALINE MINERAL CONTENT OF COMMON FLAVORING AGENTS AND CONDIMENTS (PER TABLESPOON)

Food	pH	Calcium	Magnesium	Potassium	Sodium
Lemon juice	2.2–2.6	2 mg	1 mg	15 mg	3 mg
Lime juice	2.2–2.4	1 mg	1 mg	17 mg	0 mg
Cider vinegar	2.4–3.4	0.8 mg	3 mg	14 mg	trace
Blackstrap molasses	5.0–5.4	137 mg	52mg	585 mg	19 mg
Tahini (sesame paste)	>6.0	64 mg	14 mg	110 mg	17 mg
Flax meal	>6.0	35 mg	63 mg	120 mg	7 mg
Kelp	Not available	156 mg	104 mg	753 mg	42 mg

(*Source:* Chemistry of Success.)

Can Vinegar Cure Arthritis?

Veteran international vinegar consultant Lawrence Diggs is also not convinced that vinegar is everything it's cracked up to be. "One of the persistent rumors about vinegar is that it will cure arthritis," he says. Some people believe apple cider vinegar thins body fluids. As a result, stiff joints are supposed to move easier so one won't be walking around like the Tin Man in the *Wizard of Oz*. "To date there is no scientific evidence that any kind of vinegar or vinegar cocktail will cure or relieve the pain of arthritis. I should mention also that it doesn't seem that scientists are all that interested in providing evidence either."[4]

Most doctors know it is not possible for apple cider vinegar to cure arthritis. However, because aches and pains can come and go, the healing vinegar may seem like it works wonders at times. But there is no scientific proof.

Meanwhile, if you have arthritis, watch your weight (heavy people are more at risk for osteoarthritis) by eating a low-fat diet, and get a move on. Keeping in shape can help strengthen your muscles.

Not 100% Tummy Terrific

Other people vow that vinegar is a cure-all for an upset stomach. While Vinegarman Lawrence Diggs claims he has used vinegar for himself "and it seems to have worked," he does not recommend it. "The stomach is always playing a balancing act to get the right acid and base balance. It usually doesn't get much help from us. The result is that sometimes the stomach is too base or alkaline and sometimes too acid. If it is too base then adding an acid like vinegar could help. However, if it is too acid, the problem could be made worse."

He believes because the symptoms of both conditions feel similar, we don't know if vinegar, baking soda, or burnt toast will be the best Rx. "If I had to gamble, I'd put my money on the burnt toast, even though I am not nor ever have been a member of Burnt Toast Connoisseurs International."[5]

Vinegar Remedy Flushed down the Toilet?

On May 19, 1994, a court order resulted in the destruction of 13,320 half-gallon bottles of "Jogging in a Jug"—a concoction of grape and apple juices and vinegar—because the product became an unapproved new drug due to health claims made by promoters. Jack McWilliams, owner of Third Option Laboratories, Muscle Shoals, Alabama, claimed that his vinegar solution had helped him beat arthritis and heart disease, and could lower the risk of cancer. Third Option also paid the Federal Trade Commission $480,000 to settle charges of false advertising.[6]

Meanwhile, people around the world do use healing vinegar—internally and externally—and swear that they benefit from its amazing benefits. Only you can be the judge and decide to tell if this condiment can have healing powers for you.

PART 7

VINEGAR RECIPES

Vinegar Bon Appétit!

These recipes, more than 100 mouth-watering delights, are full of nutritious fruits, vegetables, lean meats, fish, and poultry. Our tasty dishes, provided by chefs from around the country, contain a variety of vinegars—apple cider, red wine, balsamic, rice, and herbal vinegar. Plus, healthful garlic, onions, and olive oil are often part of the recipes, too.

For best results, use the vinegar brand mentioned in each recipe. However, feel free to use your own brand or a brand without sodium if so desired (because some herbal vinegars have a high sodium content).

Before you get started, I want you to first check out some must-have cooking-with-vinegar tips and pickling favorites. See how vinegars of all types can enhance immune-boosting, nutrient-rich foods. Not only will you be eating a heart-healthy, anticancer-type Mediterranean-style diet, you'll be enjoying more gusto in your meals.

VINEGAR PIZZAZZ!

Vinegar	Flavor	Uses
Apple cider vinegar	Sweet, tangy flavor	Adds golden color to sauces and marinades.
Balsamic vinegar	Sweet and flavorful	Use for special sauces, marinades or salad dressings, vanilla ice cream.
Champagne vinegar	Smooth	In sauces with poultry or seafood.
Chinese black rice vinegar	Smoky flavor	Stir-fries and salad dressings.
Garlic-flavored red wine vinegar	Zest and added zip	Excellent marinade for meats.
Malt vinegar	Hearty, deep-flavored, made from barley malt extract	Excellent on fish 'n' chips, potato salad and cole slaw, spice pickles, chutneys, relishes, in mint sauce for lamb.
Plum vinegar	Salty, citrus flavor	Salad dressings, sauces, stews, soups, and steamed vegetables.
Raspberry vinegar	Fruit flavor	Salads, vegetable dishes, marinade for chicken, blended with vanilla yogurt to make dressings for fruit salad, mixed with jam for sweet and sour sauce.
Red wine vinegar	Low-sodium, robust	Marinating dark meats, red pasta sauces, grilled steak, salad dressings.
Red wine vinegar with Italian seasoning	Flavored with oregano, garlic, onion, red pepper, and sweet basil	Salads, pasta sauces.

Vinegar	Flavor	Uses
Rice vinegar	Mild, slightly sweet	As dip for fried foods and steamed shellfish, in soups, stews, noodle dishes.
Seasoned rice vinegar	Light and zesty	Grilled chicken, cooked vegetables, green leaf salad dressing, pasta salads, quick marinade.
Sherry vinegar	Nutty flavor with a sweet aftertaste	Marinades, salad dressings, poultry dishes and tomato-based soups and sauces.
Tarragon-flavored white wine vinegar	Tasty, added zip	Excellent marinade for chicken; stir a tablespoon or so into veal recipes.
White distilled vinegar	Harsh, coarse flavor	All-purpose vinegar that can be used for a variety of kitchen and other household needs; pickling.
White rice vinegar	Pale golden color	Enhances sweet and sour dishes.
White wine vinegar	A good salt substitute	Excellent in marinades, mild salad dressings, sauces, and fish and chicken dishes.

(*Source:* Based on information provided by Four Monks Barengo [Nakano] and other sources.)

Healthful Marinating Tips

- Use red wine vinegar to marinate beef, pork, and lamb; white wine vinegar for poultry, seafood, and vegetables. Be experimental. Try tarragon white vinegar for fish; English-style malt vinegar to marinate beef or pork.
- Marinate in a nonmetallic container such as a plastic bowl, glass baking dish, or heavy-duty plastic bag.
- Marinate meat, poultry, and seafood in the refrigerator, not at room temperature.
- Pierce beef and pork several times with a fork so the marinade can seep into the meat and help tenderize it.
- *Always discard* leftover marinade used for meat, poultry, and seafood. If you want to serve some marinade on the side, it's best to make extra marinade *just* for serving.

(*Source:* Four Monks [Nakano].)

Ways to Use Vinegar

1. **Vegetables.** Liven up slightly wilted vegetables by soaking them in cold water and vinegar.

2. **Cabbage.** Add vinegar to the cooking water of boiling cabbage to prevent the odor from permeating the house.

3. **Meat.** A marinade of ½ cup of your favorite vinegar and a cup of liquid bouillon makes an effective meat tenderizer.

4. **Rice.** A tablespoon of vinegar added to the water of boiling rice makes it fluffy and white.

5. **Fish.** Reduce fishy odors by rubbing fish down with white distilled vinegar before using it.

6. **Cheese.** Keep cheese moist and fresh by wrapping it in a cloth that has been dampened with vinegar and sealing it in an airtight wrap or container.

7. **Eggs.** To produce better-formed egg whites, add a tablespoon of your favorite vinegar to the water. When boiling eggs, add some vinegar to the water to prevent the white from leaking out of a cracked egg. When poaching eggs, add a teaspoon of vinegar to the water to prevent separation.

8. **Onion Odors.** Quickly remove the odor of onions from your hands by rubbing them with distilled vinegar.

9. **Thirst Quenchers.** Mix a tablespoon of strawberry or orange vinegar in a glass filled with eight ounces of club soda and ice. It makes a delightfully cooling drink.

10. **Pickling.** Cider, red wine, balsamic, and other dark vinegars are very good for pickling, but may discolor lighter-colored pickles such as pears, onions, or cauliflowers. In this case, a distilled or white vinegar is preferred.

(*Source:* Nakano Foods, Inc., Arlington Heights, Illinois, with support from the Vinegar Institute.)

More Vinegar Moxie in the Kitchen

- Use vinegar to clean your microwave, cutting board and other kitchen equipment, and areas where you prepare food.
- Recipe calls for wine? Substitute red wine vinegar. Dilute one part of vinegar with three parts wine.
- Reduce salt. All Heinz vinegars are sodium-free, but a splash of vinegar replaces some of the salt in a recipe.
- When a recipe calls for 1 cup of buttermilk and you want a substitute, add a tablespoon of distilled white vinegar to a cup of milk instead.
- To remove pesticides from fruits and vegetables, just wash food with a mixture of 2–3 tablespoons of distilled white vinegar per quart of water.
- To keep cheese fresh and mold-free, wrap it in a cloth saturated with distilled white vinegar and store airtight in the refrigerator.
- Want gelatin recipes to hold firmer longer? Add a teaspoon of distilled white vinegar per box of gelatin to your favorite recipes. (*Source:* Heinz U.S.A.)

Pickling Passion

The Chinese invented the art of pickling, but it's the Pennsylvania Dutch who have been credited with popularizing pickling in America. Pickling is the addition of vinegar and salt—often with spices and sugar—to vegetables and fruit.

Most important, to pickle properly, vinegar is necessary to preserve food by inhibiting the growth of food-spoilage bacteria. Vinegars should be "pickling strength" (5 percent acidity), which will ensure that they are at an acidity level that is ideal for safe home preservation of foods.

According to the U.S. Department of Agriculture, the boiling-water bath method is best because it helps to kill bacteria, molds, yeast, and enzymes that spoil food.

The following hints will help you get ready for pickling and canning:

- **To Prepare:** Get a cutting board, a paring knife, standard measuring cups and spoons, a strainer or colander, and a blender, food chopper, grinder, or processor.
- **To Fill:** You'll need metal and rubber spatulas, a jar lifter, a wide-mouth funnel, a ladle with a lip, potholders, and a clean, damp cloth for wiping the jar rims before adjusting caps.
- **To Process:** You'll need a water-bath canner or a large kettle with a tight-fitting lid. The container must be deep enough for the jars to be placed on a wire rack and covered with at least 1 inch of water. Allow for enough heat space so that water doesn't boil over.
- **To Store:** Label jars with the name of the recipe and date. Store the jars in a dark, dry, cool place where they can't freeze. Beware that freezing may crack jars or break the seals, allowing bacteria to enter, which may cause spoilage.

Ten Tips for Preserving Healthy Produce

1. Select slightly underripe fruits.
2. Do not use cucumbers with a waxy surface for pickling. For best flavor and texture, pickling cucumbers should be used within 24 hours of picking.
3. Avoid soaking produce.
4. Use pure granulated pickling salt. The iodine and additives in table salt may make the pickling liquid cloudy or cause discoloration.
5. Select standard canning jars and lids. (Jars from commercially packed foods are not suitable.) Be sure jars and closures are free from nicks, chips, or cracks.
6. Never reuse canning lids; canning jars, however, may be used again.
7. Don't use copper, brass, iron, or galvanized utensils when cooking pickles. These may react with the acid and salt in the liquid and cause undesirable changes or form hazardous compounds.
8. Many recipes call for distilled white vinegar. If you prefer a fruit flavor, you may substitute apple cider vinegar.
9. Follow directions exactly; never double or triple recipes. The ratio of ingredients to vinegar may be altered, which will affect flavor and texture and may cause spoilage.
10. Use fresh spices, either whole or ground. Old spices impart a musty taste to preserved food. Cheesecloth and string work best for a "spice bag."

(*Source:* Heinz U.S.A.)

Ten Pickling Family Favorites

Apple Chutney

❖ ❖ ❖

4 pounds tart red cooking apples, cored, chopped
2 medium onions, chopped
2 cups golden raisins
1½ cups firmly packed brown sugar
1 cup Heinz Apple Cider *or* Apple Cider Flavored Vinegar
2 tablespoons grated fresh gingerroot
½ teaspoon ground mace or nutmeg
½ teaspoon salt

In a 6- to 8-quart saucepan, combine all ingredients. Bring to a boil. Reduce heat and simmer for 30–35 minutes or until thickened, stirring frequently. Immediately fill hot pint jars with mixture, leaving ½-inch headspace. Carefully run a nonmetallic utensil down side of jars to remove trapped air bubbles. Wipe jar tops and threads clean. Place hot lids on jars and screw bands on firmly. Process in boiling water canner for 10 minutes. Serve as an accompaniment to curries or beef, pork, chicken, or turkey main dishes or sandwiches. Makes 4–5 pints.

Cantaloupe Pickles

❖ ❖ ❖

4 cantaloupes (9–10 pounds), quartered, seeds and rind removed
3 cups granulated sugar
3 cups Heinz Apple Cider *or* Apple Cider Flavored Vinegar
1½ cups apple juice
6 (3-inch) cinnamon sticks, broken
2 tablespoons whole cloves
5 thin slices fresh gingerroot

Cut cantaloupe into 1-inch cubes. In a 6- to 8-quart saucepan, combine sugar, vinegar, and apple juice. Bring to a boil, stirring occasionally. Tie spices in spice bag or cheesecloth. Add spice bag to syrup and boil for 10 minutes. Add melon, reduce heat, and simmer for 15 minutes, stirring occasionally. Remove spice bag. Immediately fill hot, sterilized pint or half-pint jars with mixture, leaving ½-inch headspace. Carefully run a nonmetallic utensil down inside of jars to remove trapped air bubbles. Wipe jar tops and threads clean. Place hot lids on jars and screw bands on firmly. Process in boiling water canner—10 minutes for pints and 5 minutes for half-pints. Makes 6–7 pints or 12–14 half-pints.

Cranberry Chutney

❖ ❖ ❖

6 cups fresh cranberries (about 1½ pounds)
1½ cups Heinz Apple Cider *or* Apple Cider Flavored Vinegar
½ cup cranberry juice cocktail
1 cup granulated sugar
1 cup firmly packed brown sugar
1 cup golden raisins
2 tart apples, peeled, cored, coarsely chopped
1 orange with peel, seeded, coarsely chopped
1 medium onion, chopped
1 tablespoon chopped crystallized ginger (optional)
2 teaspoons salt
1½ teaspoons salt
½ teaspoon ground cloves or allspice
½ teaspoon red pepper

In a 6- to 8-quart saucepan, combine all ingredients. Bring to a boil. Reduce heat and simmer for 45 minutes to 1 hour or until thick. Stir occasionally at the beginning of cooking and constantly at the end of cooking. Immediately fill half-pint jars with mixture, leaving ½-inch headspace. Carefully run a nonmetallic utensil down inside of jars to remove trapped air bubbles. Wipe jar tops and threads clean. Place hot lids on jars and screw bands on firmly. Process in boiling water canner for 10 minutes. Serve as an accompaniment to curries for chicken, turkey, wild game, lamb, or beef dishes. Makes about 8 half-pints.

Cucumber Dill Relish

❖ ❖ ❖

1 tablespoon mixed pickling spice
4 pounds pickling cucumbers, chopped
2 medium onions, chopped
1 small head cabbage, chopped
3 cloves garlic, minced
2 cups Heinz Apple Cider *or* Apple Cider Flavored Vinegar
½ cup granulated sugar
2 tablespoons snipped fresh dill weed
1 tablespoon pickling salt
5–10 sprigs fresh dill weed

Tie pickling spice in a spice bag or cheesecloth. In a 6- to 8-quart saucepan, combine spice bag and remaining ingredients except dill sprigs. Mix well. Bring to a boil over medium-high heat, stirring occasionally. Reduce heat to medium and cook for 15 minutes, stirring frequently. Remove spice bag. Immediately fill hot pint or half-pint jars with mixture, leaving ½-inch headspace. Place 1–2 sprigs of dill weed on top of mixture. Carefully run a nonmetallic utensil down side of jars to remove trapped air bubbles. Wipe jar tops and threads clean. Place hot lids on jars and screw bands on firmly. Process pints or half-pints in boiling water canner 15 minutes. Makes 5–6 pints or 10–12 half-pints.

Green Tomato Relish

❖ ❖ ❖

6 pounds green tomatoes, chopped
2 large red bell peppers (about 1 pound), chopped
2 large green bell peppers (about1 pound), chopped
2 medium onions, chopped
¼ cup pickling salt
2 tablespoons mustard seed
2 tablespoons celery seed
1 tablespoon mixed pickling spice
4 cups Heinz Apple Cider *or* Apple Cider Flavored Vinegar
2 cups firmly packed brown sugar

In a large bowl, combine tomatoes, peppers, and onions. Sprinkle with pickling salt and mix well. Cover and chill overnight. Drain well. Tie mustard seed, celery seed, and pickling spice in a spice bag or cheesecloth. In a 6- to 8-quart saucepan, combine vegetables, vinegar, sugar, and spice bag. Bring to a boil over medium heat, stirring occasionally. Reduce heat and simmer for 30 minutes, stirring often to prevent sticking. Remove spice bag. Immediately fill hot pint or half-pint jars with mixture, leaving ½-inch headspace. Carefully run a nonmetallic utensil down inside of jars to remove trapped air bubbles. Wipe jar tops and threads clean. Place hot lids on jars and screw bands on firmly. Process pints or half-pints in boiling water canner for 15 minutes. Makes 6–7 pints or 12–14 half-pints.

End-of-the Garden Pickles

6 cups Heinz Distilled White Vinegar
4 cups granulated sugar
1½ cups water
3 tablespoons mixed pickling spice
2 tablespoons pickling salt
3 cups broccoli flowerets
3 cups caulifloweretes
3 cups carrot pieces (about 1-inch)
3 cups cubed unpeeled cucumber (about 1-inch)
3 cups zucchini chunks (about 1-inch)
2 cups red or green bell pepper squares (about 1-inch)
2 medium onions, each cut into eight wedges

In an 8- to 10-quart saucepan, combine vinegar, sugar, water, pickling spice, and salt. Bring to a boil, stirring occasionally. Boil for 4 minutes. Add vegetables, reduce heat, and simmer until vegetables are hot, about 5 minutes. Immediately fill hot quart jars with mixture, leaving ½-inch headspace. Carefully run a nonmetallic utensil down side of jars to remove trapped air bubbles. Wipe jar tops and threads clean. Place hot lids on jars and screw bands on firmly. Process in boiling water canner for 15 minutes. Makes about 4 quarts.

Garlic Dill Pickles

❖ ❖ ❖

4 pounds (3- to 4-inch) pickling cucumbers
6 cups water
4½ cups Heinz Apple Cider *or* Apple Cider Flavored Vinegar
6 tablespoons pickling salt
¾ teaspoon of crushed red pepper (optional)
16 cloves garlic, split
16 heads fresh dill

Wash cucumbers and remove 1/16-inch from the blossom end. In a 3-quart saucepan, combine water, vinegar, salt, and red pepper. Bring to a boil. Meanwhile, place 2 pieces of garlic and 1 head of dill in each hot pint jar. Firmly pack cucumbers upright in jars, leaving ½-inch headspace. Place 2 additional pieces of garlic and 1 head of dill in each hot pint jar. Immediately pour hot vinegar mixture over cucumbers, leaving ½-inch headspace. Carefully run a nonmetallic utensil down side of jars to remove trapped air bubbles. Wipe jar tops and threads clean. Place hot lids on jars and screw bands on firmly. Process in boiling water canner for 10 minutes. Makes about 7–8 pints.

Pineapple Raisin Sauce

❖ ❖ ❖

4 cans (20 ounces each) crushed pineapple in unsweetened juice, undrained
3 cups firmly packed brown sugar
2 cups Heinz Apple Cider *or* Apple Cider Flavored Vinegar
2 cups raisins
1 cup chopped onions
3 tablespoons grated orange peel
3 tablespoons Dijon-style mustard
2 tablespoons soy sauce

In a 6-quart saucepan, combine all ingredients. Bring to a boil, stirring occasionally. Reduce heat and simmer about 45 minutes or until there is just a small amount of liquid remaining. Immediately fill hot pint jars with mixture, leaving ½-inch headspace. Carefully run a nonmetallic utensil down inside of jars to remove trapped air bubbles. Wipe jar tops and threads clean. Place hot lids on jars and screw bands on firmly. Process in boiling water canner for 10 minutes. Serve as an accompaniment to pork, ham, turkey, or chicken main dishes or sandwiches. Makes about 6 pints.

Summer Squash Relish

❖ ❖ ❖

10 cups chopped zucchini and yellow summer squash (about 10–12 medium)
1 medium onion, chopped
1 medium red bell pepper, chopped
1 medium green bell pepper, chopped
2 cups Heinz Apple Cider *or* Apple Cider Flavored Vinegar
2½ cups granulated sugar
2 teaspoons mustard seed
2 teaspoons celery seed
2 teaspoons ground cinnamon
2 teaspoons tumeric
1 teaspoon pickling salt

In a 6- to 8-quart saucepan, combine all ingredients. Bring to a boil over medium-high heat, stirring occasionally. Reduce heat and simmer for 10 minutes or until thickened, stirring frequently. Immediately fill hot pint or half-pint jars with mixture, leaving ½-inch headspace. Carefully run a nonmetallic utensil down inside of jars to remove trapped air bubbles. Wipe jar tops and threads clean. Place lids on jars and screw bands on firmly. Process pints or half-pints in boiling water canner for 15 minutes. Makes 5–6 pints or 10–12 half-pints.

Zucchini Pickles

❖ ❖ ❖

2 pounds zucchini
¼ cup pickling salt
6 cups water
1 package (16 ounces) frozen pearl onions, thawed
3 *cups* Heinz Apple Cider *or* Apple Cider Flavored Vinegar
2 cups firmly packed brown sugar
1 tablespoon mustard seed
1 tablespoon tumeric
1½ teaspoons ground ginger

Wash zucchini and cut into 3x½-inch pieces. In a large bowl, combine zucchini, salt, and water. Mix well. Cover and let stand for 2 hours. Drain and rinse well. In a 6- to 8-quart saucepan, combine zucchini, onions, and remaining ingredients. Bring to a boil over medium-high heat, stirring occasionally. Boil for 5 minutes, stirring constantly. Immediately fill hot pint jars with zucchini and onions, leaving ½-inch headspace. Immediately pour hot vinegar mixture over zucchini, maintaining ½-inch headspace. Carefully run a nonmetallic utensil down inside of jars to remove trapped air bubbles. Wipe jar tops and threads clean. Place hot lids on jars and screw bands on firmly. Process in boiling water canner for 15 minutes. Makes about 4–5 pints.

Sweet Vinegar Fact

Most vinegars will last for at least one or two years—if unopened. However, fruit vinegars do not keep as long as other vinegars.

Vinegar Substitutions

Although our chefs suggest specific flavored vinegars in some of these recipes, if you are on a low-sodium diet, try the dish with a plain vinegar such as apple cider, red wine, rice, or balsamic. Also, if you don't have the brand of vinegar or olive oil called for in these recipes, substitute a similar type for best results.

The Vinegar Health-Boosting Five-Day Menu Plan

* Recipes appear below.

Day 1

Breakfast

1 tablespoon *each* of vinegar
and honey in 6-ounce glass of water (optional)
(apple cider vinegar)

Low-Fat Raspberry and Yogurt Dressing* with waffles
(raspberry vinegar)

1 cup fresh-squeezed orange juice

Lunch

Tossed Chef's Salad* *(seasoned red wine vinegar)*

1 cup skim milk

Snack

1 bowl Gazpacho* *(red wine vinegar)*

4 low-sodium whole wheat crackers

Dinner

1 serving Hearty Garlic Chili* *(red wine vinegar)*

1 serving Steamed Artichokes with Yogurt
and Buttermilk Dressing* *(seasoned rice vinegar with basil and oregano)*

cornbread with 1 teaspoon honey

Snack

1 cup Melon Sorbet* *(white wine vinegar)*

Day 2

Breakfast

1 tablespoon *each* of vinegar
and honey in 6-ounce glass of water (optional)
(apple cider vinegar)

1 serving Strawberries with Orange and Balsamic Vinegar* *(balsamic vinegar)*

2/3 cup oatmeal and 1/2 teaspoon nutmeg
1/2 cup skim milk

Lunch

Pasta Primavera Salad* *(seasoned apple cider vinegar)*
1 fresh apple
1 cup skim milk

Snack

Chicken Bite Appetizers* *(red wine vinegar)*

Dinner

Simple Salmon* *(red wine vinegar)*
Garden Vegetable Potpourri* *(seasoned apple cider vinegar)*
Focaccia dipped in olive oil

Snack

Low-fat Mango and Vanilla Yogurt Dressing* with 1–1 1/2 cups fresh fruit *(mango vinegar)*

Day 3

Breakfast

2–3 tablespoons Nonfat Yogurt Cheese* *(apple cider vinegar)* spread on 1 cinnamon-raisin bagel
3/4 cup bran flakes with 1/2 cup skim milk
1/2 pink grapefruit

Lunch

Tofu and Toasted Peanut Salad* *(seasoned rice vinegar)*
fresh bakery sourdough bread dipped in olive oil
1 cup skim milk

Snack

1 cup Cold Fresh Vegetable Soup* *(red wine vinegar)*

Dinner

Mediterranean Steamed Chicken* *(red wine vinegar)*
Baked Sweet Potatoes with

Plantain and Citrus Chutney* *(rice vinegar)*
tossed green salad *(balsamic vinaigrette)*

Snack
1 piece Old-Fashioned Raisin Pie* *(vinegar)*

Day 4

Breakfast
1 tablespoon *each* of vinegar and honey in 6 ounces water (optional) *(apple cider vinegar)*
scrambled eggs
2 slices whole wheat toast
6 ounces unsweetened grapefruit juice

Lunch
Chinese Chicken Salad* *(white wine vinegar)*
herbal tea
1 slice sourdough bread dipped in olive oil

Snack
1 orange

Dinner
Mediterranean Beef Stew* *(seasoned rice vinegar)*
tossed green salad with Vinaigrette*

Snack
Pound cake topped with Low-fat Peach and Vanilla Yogurt Dressing* *(peach vinegar)*

Day 5

Breakfast
whole wheat pancakes with blueberry syrup
fresh-squeezed orange juice
herbal tea

Lunch

Venetian Pasta Salad* *(seasoned red wine vinegar)*

Snack

red grapes

Dinner

Stir-Fry Shrimp and Rice* *(rice vinegar)*
Marinated Green Vegetables* *(red wine vinegar)*

Snack

vanilla ice cream with 1 tablespoon of vinegar drizzled on top *(balsamic vinegar)*

Soups

It's smart to go for good nutrition and filling, low-fat satisfaction. And these healthful soups offer just that.

Studies show that soup is particularly effective in filling you up, so a bowl of soup before a meal can take the edge off your appetite. And because it's eaten spoonful by spoonful, you'll eat it slowly, which gives your brain time to register that you're getting full.

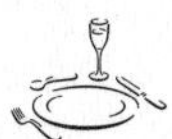

Cold Gold Soup
Court Bouillon
Gazpacho
Hot and Sour Soup

Cold Gold Soup

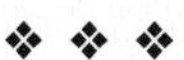

3 large peaches, ripe
2 teaspoons honey
½ cup orange juice, fresh squeezed
2 drops Tabasco sauce
white pepper
1 tablespoon balsamic vinegar
1 tablespoon mint, finely chopped
orange peel

Peel peaches and cut into small chunks. Add honey and orange juice. Blend until smooth. Stir in Tabasco and white pepper, cover, and chill at least 1 hour.

Stir in vinegar and chopped mint, then ladle soup into chilled bowls. Garnish with fresh whole mint leaves and zests of orange peel. Serves 3.

(Courtesy of *Amazing Apple Cider Vinegar* by Earl L. Mindell with Larry M. Johns.)

Court Bouillon

❖ ❖ ❖

Court bouillon is a very nice liquid for poaching fish and/or vegetables. It is very simple to make and will keep nicely in the refrigerator for 10 days.

2½ quarts cold water
5 ounces apple cider vinegar or white wine vinegar
1 teaspoon salt
6 ounces carrots, sliced
8 ounces onions, sliced
pinch thyme, whole, dried
3 or 4 parsley stems
2 bay leaves
¼ ounce peppercorns, whole

Combine all ingredients except peppercorns and simmer for 45 minutes. Add the peppercorns and simmer for 15 more minutes. Cool and refrigerate for later use. This recipe makes ½ gallon.

(Recipe by Chef Salvatore J. Campagna.)

Gazpacho
Cold Fresh Vegetable Soup

❖ ❖ ❖

1 pound tomato concasse (recipe below)
8 ounces onions, peeled, sliced
8 ounces red bell peppers, seeded, quartered
8 ounces cucumbers, seeded, quartered
1 tablespoon garlic, minced
3 ounces red wine vinegar
Juice of 2 lemons
3 ounces olive oil
Juice of 2 limes
1 teaspoon salt
Tabasco, habanero (new) to taste
16 ounces tomato juice

Tomato Concasse

Cut out the stems of 4 tomatoes (1 pound) and cut a small "x" on the bottom of each one. Place tomatoes in boiling water for 15–30 seconds, depending on ripeness. Remove tomatoes with slotted spoon and immediately plunge into ice water and gently pull away the skin. Cut tomatoes in half and squeeze out the seeds and dice. For added flavor, sauté diced tomatoes in 2 ounces of olive oil with a teaspoon of chopped garlic. Set aside to cool.

Puree all ingredients except the tomato juice. Adjust the consistency and flavor with the tomato juice (or consommé). Adjust seasoning with salt and pepper and garnish with a very small dice of red and green bell pepper, cucumber, and tomato along with small seasoned croutons. A teaspoon of the diced vegetables and a few croutons are ideal. Makes ½ gallon.

(Recipe by Chef Salvatore J. Campagna.)

Hot and Sour Soup

❖ ❖ ❖

1 (32-ounce) carton chicken broth or 4 cups homemade or canned chicken broth

3 tablespoons Nakano Natural Rice Vinegar *or* Nakano Seasoned Rice Vinegar—Original

2 tablespoons lite or regular soy sauce

¼ teaspoon crushed red pepper flakes or 1 teaspoon hot chile oil

4 ounces firm silken tofu, well drained*

1 (15-ounce) can stir-fry mushrooms or 2 jars (7 ounces each) straw mushrooms, drained

½ cup julienned canned bamboo shoots

3 tablespoons water

2 tablespoons cornstarch

1 egg white, slightly beaten

¼ cup thinly sliced green onions

2 teaspoons dark roasted sesame oil

Combine broth, vinegar, soy sauce, and pepper flakes in a large saucepan; bring to a boil over high heat. Reduce heat to medium; simmer 2 minutes. Stir in tofu, mushrooms, and bamboo shoots; heat through. Combine water and cornstarch, mixing until smooth. Stir into soup; cook until soup boils and thickens, about 5 minutes, stirring frequently. Turn off heat under saucepan. Stirring soup constantly in one direction, slowly pour egg white in a thin stream into soup. Stir in green onions and sesame oil. Ladle into soup bowls. Serves 4 (makes about 5½ cups).

*Tip: Look for silken tofu in the produce section of your supermarket. If it is not available, you may use 1 cup diced cooked chicken or pork.

Salads

A salad should have plenty of fresh vegetables and fruits. To enhance its flavor and its nutrients, what better way than to top it off with vinegar. Whether it's apple cider, red wine, rice, balsamic or herbal vinegars, you can count on a salad being a healthful side dish or complete meal.

Combine olive oil, garlic, and onions—which many of these salads contain—and you've got a wholesome, nutritious dish.

Antipasto Appetizer Salad
Apple-Pecan Spinach Salad
Avocado and Romaine Salad with Raspberry-Raspberry Vinaigrette
Chinese Chicken Salad
Fast Fabulous Coleslaw
Five-Bean Salad
Green Bean and Mushroom Salad
Green Bean and Red Potato Salad
Greek Salad with Spiced Onions
Indian Summer Potato Salad
Mediterranean Red Potato Salad
Raspberry, Blue Cheese, and Toasted Walnut Salad
Raspberry Three-Bean Salad
Santa Fe Rice Salad
Spinach Salad
Tofu and Toasted Peanut Salad
Tossed Chef's Salad
Tropical Fruit Salad with Fruit Vinaigrette

Antipasto Appetizer Salad

Prepare 1 quart of any of the selected vegetables, etc., listed:

cauliflower flowerets
whole fresh mushrooms
cherry tomatoes
sweet red pepper squares
celery, cut into 1-inch pieces
garbanzo beans
kidney beans
red onion wedges
pitted ripe olives
canned artichoke hearts in water
Spanish olives, stuffed with anchovies
cubes of mozzarella or Monterey Jack cheese
½ cup Nakano Italian Seasoned Red Wine Vinegar
pinch black pepper

Cauliflower should be precooked in boiling water only 3 minutes and mushrooms only 1 minute; drain immediately. Poke cherry tomatoes with a thin toothpick four times. Combine cheese and all vegetables except red pepper, and spread in a thin layer in a flat glass baking dish. Pour vinegar over top. Sprinkle with pepper. Stir vegetables frequently while marinating a half hour or longer. Drain before serving. Serves 12.

Apple-Pecan Spinach Salad

3 tablespoons Four Monks Red Wine Vinegar
1 clove garlic, finely chopped
½ teaspoon salt
⅛ teaspoon pepper
1 egg beaten
⅓ cup vegetable oil
4 cups lightly packed spinach leaves
⅔ cup pecan halves, toasted
⅔ cup diced red apple

Combine vinegar and next 4 ingredients. Whisk in oil. Toss dressing with spinach, pecans, and apples. Serves 6.

Avocado and Romaine Salad with Raspberry-Raspberry Vinaigrette

❖ ❖ ❖

1 cup fresh raspberries
¼ cup Spectrum Naturals Organic Raspberry Wine Vinegar
2 small heads romaine lettuce, washed, dried
2 ripe avocados, peeled and sliced
½ cup Spectrum Naturals Pure Pressed Canola Oil (or Spectrum Naturals Super Canola Oil)
2 teaspoons fresh tarragon, minced (optional)
¾ teaspoon salt
fresh ground pepper to taste

In a small mixing bowl, combine raspberries and vinegar. Mash berries and allow them to soak in the vinegar while preparing the lettuce and avocados. Whisk canola oil into the berry/vinegar mixture, add tarragon, salt, and pepper. Arrange the lettuce and avocados attractively in a salad bowl. Spoon 6 or 8 tablespoons of the vinaigrette over the salad and serve immediately. The remaining dressing will keep for 2–3 days in the refrigerator.

(Recipe created by Chef Gary Jenanyan.)

Chinese Chicken Salad

❖ ❖ ❖

Now you can make this popular restaurant dish at home! For added flavor, season uncooked chicken with salt and sprinkle generously with sesame seeds. Sauté in peanut oil; cool before slicing or shredding.

Crystallized ginger is available in the spice or ethnic food sections of supermarkets, and in Asian food stores.

3 *tablespoons* Nakano White Wine Vinegar
1 tablespoon each soy sauce and honey
2 teaspoons sesame oil
2–3 boneless, skinless chicken breast halves, cooked and sliced
8 cups coarsely shredded iceberg lettuce (approx. 1 medium head)
½ cup chopped cilantro
⅓ cup chopped roasted peanuts
¼ cup sliced green onions
¼ cup chopped crystallized ginger

In a small bowl, combine vinegar, soy sauce, honey, and sesame oil. In a large bowl, combine remaining ingredients. Toss with dressing and serve immediately. Serves 4–6.

Fast Fabulous Coleslaw

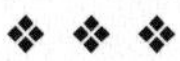

Salad

4 cups green cabbage, thinly shredded and packed in cup
1½ cups red cabbage, thinly shredded and packed in cup
1 cup carrots, finely grated
1 cup red pepper, minced
Vidalia or red onion (optional)
fresh dill, minced

Dressing

1 cup Spectrum Naturals Canola Mayonnaise
2 tablespoons Spectrum Naturals Apple Cider Vinegar
1 tablespoon maple syrup
1 tablespoon celery seed
salt and pepper to taste

Prepare vegetables for salad. Combine carrots, red peppers, onion, and dill in a large bowl. Whisk together dressing ingredients and pour over vegetables, toss gently. Serve immediately or refrigerate until ready to enjoy.

(Recipe created by Helen Pimentel of Bread & Circus.)

Five-Bean Salad

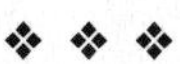

16-ounce can (2 cups) green and wax cut beans, drained (fresh beans may be substituted—1 cup each)
8-ounce can (1 cup) garbanzo beans, drained and rinsed
8-ounce can (1 cup) pinto beans, drained and rinsed
½ cup Nakano Seasoned Rice Vinegar with Red Pepper
½ cup chopped green pepper
¼ cup chopped red onion

Combine all ingredients in large salad bowl. Refrigerate 1 hour or longer, stirring several times to blend flavors. Serves 9.

Green Bean and Mushroom Salad

1½ pounds green beans, fresh
1¼ pounds button mushrooms, fresh
4 ounces extra virgin olive oil
2 ounces red wine vinegar
salt to taste
freshly ground pepper to taste
1 large head Romaine lettuce
2 large tomatoes, ripe

Wash and clean green beans. Boil in 2 quarts of salted water until tender and immediately immerse in an ice bath. When cool, cut beans into 2- to 3-inch lengths. Set aside to dry on paper towels. Wash button mushrooms gently under cold running water. Cut into ¼-inch slices. Marinate mushroom slices in large bowl with two ounces of oil and 1 ounce of red wine vinegar with a little salt and pepper. Wash and dry Romaine lettuce leaves. Discard outer leaves, saving lighter green leaves. Break into small bite-size pieces and place in large salad bowl. Add green beans to mushroom bowl and toss lightly. Pour marinade from green beans and mushrooms onto lettuce and toss. Add a little more oil if necessary. Now add 2 ounces of oil and 1 ounce of vinegar to green beans and mushrooms and toss. Taste for salt and pepper and adjust if necessary. Cut each tomato into 6 wedges. Place 2 wedges of tomato and a portion of lettuce on a cold plate. Place the marinated green beans and mushrooms on top of the lettuce and serve immediately. Serves 6.

(Recipe by Chef Salvatore J. Campagna.)

Green Bean and Red Potato Salad

❖ ❖ ❖

1 pound small red potatoes
8 ounces fresh green beans
1 cup sliced celery
¼ cup chopped green onions
½ cup Nakano Seasoned Apple Cider Vinegar
1 teaspoon Dijon mustard
¼ teaspoon each dill weed and celery salt
pinch black pepper

Cook whole potatoes 20 minutes. Trim ends of fresh beans and cut in half. Add beans to potatoes and cook together for about 10 minutes or until potatoes are cooked but firm. Drain and cool. Cut potatoes into pieces, leaving red skin. Toss potatoes and beans with celery and onions. Combine vinegar with remaining ingredients and toss with salad. Chill an hour longer. Serves 6.

Greek Salad with Spice Onions

❖ ❖ ❖

6 cups thinly sliced red onions
3 (3-inch) cinnamon sticks, broken in half
8 whole cloves
2 cups water
1½ cups cider vinegar
1 cup sugar
Greek salad (see instructions)

Combine all ingredients except Greek salad in a saucepan. Cover, bring to boil, then simmer for 5 minutes. Cool in liquid. Drain liquid and discard cinnamon. Chill in closed container.

To make Greek salad: Line platter with 4 cups of dark green lettuces. Top with 2 tomatoes, sliced; 1 cucumber, sliced; and 1 cup spiced onions. Sprinkle with 2 tablespoons chopped mint and cracked pepper to taste. For dressing, combine 2 tablespoons olive oil and juice from 2 fresh lemons. Drizzle over salad. Makes 4 servings.

(Recipe created by the National Onion Association.)

Indian Summer Potato Salad

❖ ❖ ❖

1 pound red potatoes, cooked
½ cup chopped onions
¼ cup Nakano Seasoned Rice Vinegar
½ teaspoon salt
½ teaspoon dill weed
⅛ teaspoon white pepper
⅓ cup light mayonnaise
1 teaspoon mustard
½ cup frozen peas
1 cup sliced celery
1 cup tart red apple wedges

Peel potatoes while still warm and cut into wedges; place in large bowl with onions. (For milder flavor, cook onions with potatoes the last 2 minutes.) Pour vinegar, salt, dill weed, and pepper over potatoes to marinate until cool. Blend mayonnaise with mustard; mix with potatoes. Rinse peas in boiling water. Fold peas, celery, and apples into salad. Refrigerate salad for at least an hour. Best served same day. Makes eight ½-cup servings.

Mediterranean Red Potato Salad

❖ ❖ ❖

8 medium-size red potatoes, quartered
½ cup Spectrum Naturals Organic Extra Virgin Olive Oil
¼ cup Spectrums Naturals Organic Italian Herb Wine Vinegar
2 tablespoons Spectrum World Cuisine Mediterranean Seasoning Oil
2 shallots, finely minced
¼ cup fresh basil, chopped
¼ cup fresh parsley, chopped
salt and fresh ground pepper to taste

Place the potatoes in a large saucepan. Cover with cool water. Bring to a boil and simmer until done, about 20 minutes. Meanwhile, in a large bowl, combine olive oil, vinegar, seasoning oil, and shallots. When potatoes are done, drain water and transfer to oil and vinegar mixture. Toss well. Add herbs, season with salt and pepper. Let stand a few minutes, toss again, and correct the seasoning. May be served warm or cold with roasted or grilled meats, poultry, or fish.

Raspberry, Blue Cheese, and Toasted Walnut Salad

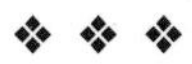

2 shallots, finely chopped
1 tablespoon Bread & Circus Dijon Mustard
2 tablespoons Spectrum Naturals Balsamic Vinegar
¼ cup Spectrum Naturals Organic Raspberry Wine Vinegar
2 tablespoons honey
1 tablespoon fresh orange juice
1 cup Spectrum Naturals Organic Extra Virgin Olive Oil
¼ cup walnuts
2 cups baby lettuce mixture
1 cup fresh raspberries
2 ounces Danish Blue or Roquefort cheese

In medium bowl, combine shallots and mustard with vinegar. Add honey and orange juice: whisk to blend. Drizzle in olive oil. Toast walnuts in shallow pan at 350° for 15 minutes. Let cool and roughly chop. In large bowl, toss lettuce mix with raspberries and ½ cup vinaigrette to taste. Divide greens on four plates and top with crumbled blue cheese and walnuts.

(Recipe adapted from: *Berries*, *A Country Garden Cookbook*, by Sharon Kramis.)

Raspberry Three-Bean Salad

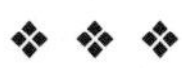

1 8-ounce can each red, garbanzo, and black beans, drained
¼ cup Spectrum Naturals Extra Virgin Olive Oil (or Certified Organic Extra Virgin, Imported Extra Virgin, or Californian Extra Virgin Olive Oil)
3 green onions, chopped
2 tablespoons cilantro, chopped
2 carrots, chopped
½ green bell pepper, chopped
½ red bell pepper, chopped
1 cup waxed or green beans, lightly steamed
salt and fresh ground pepper to taste

Combine all ingredients and chill overnight. Serves 4–6.

Santa Fe Rice Salad

❖ ❖ ❖

2 cups chilled cooked white rice
¾ cup rinsed and drained canned black beans or kidney beans
1 large tomato, seeded, diced
¾ cup diced sharp Cheddar cheese
⅓ cup sliced green onions
⅓ cup vegetable oil
¼ cup Nakano Seasoned Rice Vinegar with Roasted Garlic *or* Nakano Seasoned Rice Vinegar—Original
*1 tablespoon minced canned chipotle chilies in adobo sauce or bottled or fresh minced jalapeño peppers**
½ teaspoon sugar
1 small ripe avocado, peeled, seeded, diced

In a large bowl, combine rice, beans, tomato, cheese, and green onions; mix well. In a small bowl, combine remaining ingredients except avocado; mix well. Pour over rice mixture; mix well. Cover and refrigerate at least 30 minutes or up to 24 hours before serving. Just before serving, stir in avocado. Serve chilled or at room temperature. Makes about 5 cups. Serves 6.

*Tip: Look for bottled minced jalapeño chili peppers in the produce section of your supermarket next to the bottled minced garlic.

Spinach Salad

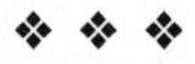

½ cup blueberry vinegar
1 tablespoon brown sugar
2 teaspoons Worcestershire
dash of Tabasco
½ cup crisp bacon bits
¼ cup olive oil
2 teaspoons oil
2 bunches spinach, stemmed and washed

Heat pan, add vinegar, and reduce to 50 percent. Add sugar and melt. Add Worchestershire, Tabasco, bacon, and oil. Heat, pour over spinach, and toss.

(Recipe created by Valley View Blueberries.)

Tofu and Toasted Peanut Salad

8 ounces firm tofu, cut into ½-inch cubes
½ cup lightly salted roast peanuts
½ cup diced celery
½ cup diced green bell pepper
2 tablespoons lite soy sauce
2 tablespoons Nakano Seasoned Rice Vinegar—Original *or* Nakano Seasoned Rice Vinegar with Red Pepper
2 teaspoons dark roasted sesame oil
2 teaspoons peanut or vegetable oil
1 teaspoon honey
1 green onion, minced
salt and ground white pepper
1 small head napa or Chinese cabbage, finely shredded
¼ cup chopped fresh cilanto or 1 green onion, thinly sliced

Place tofu, peanuts, celery, and green pepper in a medium bowl. Combine soy sauce, vinegar, sesame oil, peanut oil and honey; mix until honey dissolves. Stir in minced green onion; mix well. Pour dressing over tofu mixture. Season with salt and pepper to taste. Divide cabbage among 4 plates. Spoon tofu mixture equally over cabbage. Garnish with cilantro or onion. Serves 4.

Tossed Chef's Salad

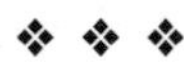

1 head iceberg lettuce, cut into cubes or 2 heads red butter lettuce, torn into pieces
4 ounces low-fat turkey ham, cut into strips
4 ounces low-fat cheddar cheese
4 ounces cooked chicken breast, cut into strips
2 Italian pear-shaped tomatoes, diced
¼ cup sliced radishes
1 tablespoon sliced chives or green onion
½ cup Nakano Light French Dressing Seasoned with Red Wine Vinegar

In a large salad bowl, combine all ingredients. Toss with dressing just before serving. Serves 4.

Tropical Fruit Salad with Fruit Vinaigrette

❖ ❖ ❖

1 ripe papaya, seeded, peeled, and diced
1 ripe mango, peeled, pitted, and diced
2 kiwi fruit, peeled and sliced
2 cups diced fresh pineapple
¾ cup Nakano Seasoned Rice Vinegar
2 tablespoons chopped red onion
1 tablespoon honey
¼ teaspoon allspice
½ cup vegetable oil
salt and ground white pepper to taste
1 ripe medium banana
1 cup sliced strawberries
2 teaspoon chopped fresh mint leaves
¼ cup shredded sweetened coconut, toasted (optional)

Place half of papaya, mango, kiwi fruit, and pineapple in a small nonaluminum saucepan. Combine remaining papaya, mango, kiwi fruit, and pineapple in a medium bowl; cover and refrigerate. Add vinegar to fruit in saucepan; cook over medium heat 5 minutes or until fruit is softened. Transfer to refrigerator; chill 30 minutes. Pour vinegar mixture into a food processor or blender; add onion, honey, and allspice. Process until mixture is smooth. With motor running, pour oil through feed tube in a steady stream. Process just until well blended. Season with salt and pepper. Add banana, strawberries, and mint to reserved fruit; toss lightly. Add ½ cup dressing, toss again. Spoon into serving dishes; sprinkle with toasted coconut, if desired. Serves 6.

Remaining dressing may be refrigerated up to 1 week. Use as a marinade for chicken or pork or as a dressing on a mixed green salad with sliced ripe avocado and grapefruit sections.

Dressings—Sauces—Spreads

Dressings and sauces to accompany healing foods can be just more healthful ingredients—especially when they include vinegar, olive oil, and herbs. Not only will you enjoy the nutritious benefits of these recipes, but the Mediterranean flair and flavor are a health bonus.

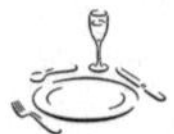

Basil and Spinach Pesto
Cool Fruit Salad Dressing
Creamy Caesar-Style Dressing
Easy Balsamic Vinaigrette or Marinade
Eggless Provençale Rouille
Garlic and Herb Dressing
Honey Miso Sauce
Honey Sherry Dressing
Make-Your-Own-Salsa
Nonfat Yogurt Cheese
New-Wave Italian Meat Sauce
Silken Tofu Tartare Sauce
Sweet and Sour Mustard Dipping Sauce
Quick Two-Tomato Sauce with Black Olives
Vinaigrette Sauce for Vegetables
Wine Butter Sauce for Fish

Basil and Spinach Pesto

❖ ❖ ❖

1 bunch basil
1 bunch fresh spinach
5 cloves garlic
6 tablespoons Spectrum Naturals Tuscan Style Extra Virgin Olive Oil
6 tablespoons Spectrum Essentials Hemp Oil
¼ cup Parmesan cheese
¼ cup toasted walnuts
salt and pepper

In a blender, combine half the greens and all of the garlic. Add half of the oil and blend until pureed. Add the rest of the greens, a handful at a time, adding oil as needed. Add the cheese and walnuts and continue to puree. Season with salt and pepper. Pesto can be stored for 2 weeks covered in the refrigerator or frozen up to 6 months.

Since this recipe contains hemp oil, a fragile nutritional oil, the pesto should not be used over high heat. It may be added to hot pastas, soups, sauces, and salads. This recipe may also be changed to use a total of ¾ cup Spectrum Naturals Organic Olive Oil in place of hemp oil. Makes approximately 1½ cups.

(Recipe created by Chef Gary Jenanyan.)

Cool Fruit Salad Dressing

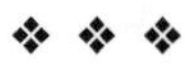

2 tablespoons Pompeian Pure *or* Extra Light Olive Oil
2 tablespoons Pompeian Red Wine Vinegar
1 teaspoon sugar
2 tablespoons mint leaves, chopped
½ cup sour cream (or light substitute
1 tablespoon lemon juice
1 tablespoon ground cumin
2 tablespoons fresh cilantro, chopped

Combine all ingredients, mix well, and chill thoroughly. Toss with your favorite seasonal salad ingredients such as apples, bananas, and citrus. Serve at once.

Creamy Caesar-Style Dressing

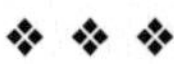

3 large garlic cloves, peeled, halved
2 teaspoons salt
4 anchovy fillets
1 teaspoon dry mustard
2 teaspoons Worcestershire sauce
2 tablespoons fresh lemon juice
2½ tablespoons red wine vinegar
¾ cup olive oil
1 egg, well beaten

Place the garlic in the work bowl of a food processor fitted with the steel blade and mince it. Add the salt, anchovy fillets, and dry mustard. Process 10 seconds. Add the Worcestershire sauce, lemon juice, and red wine vinegar and process 10 seconds. With the machine running, slowly add all the olive oil, then drizzle in the egg until a creamy emulsion has formed. Refrigerate. Let dressing stand half an hour at room temperature before tossing with greens. The dressing will keep refrigerated for about 5 days.

(Indian Summer, Inc.)

Easy Balsamic Vinaigrette or Marinade

8 *tablespoons* Spectrum Naturals Extra Virgin Olive Oil
2 *tablespoons* Spectrum Naturals Balsamic Vinegar
2 teaspoons chives, minced
2 teaspoons parsley, minced
2 teaspoons thyme, minced
salt and pepper to taste

Serve over your favorite salad or marinate fish, chicken, or beef. For a variation, add 2 teaspoons Dijon-style mustard.

(Recipe by Chef Gary Jenanyan.)

Eggless Provençale Rouille (Hot Pepper Sauce)

❖ ❖ ❖

2 tablespoons Spectrum Naturals California Extra Virgin Olive Oil *(or* Certified Organic Extra Virgin, Imported Extra Virgin*)*
10-oz tub Spectrum Spread *(a healthful butter and margarine substitute, no trans-fatty acids)*
1 large red bell pepper, roasted, peeled, seeded, and finely diced (jarred variety works well for this recipe)
2 tablespoons fresh garlic, very finely minced
1 pinch saffron, optional
2 teaspoons salt
fresh ground pepper to taste

In a stainless steel or glass bowl, whisk olive oil into Spectrum Spread. Stir in peppers and garlic. Stir in saffron. Season with salt and pepper. Cover and refrigerate until ready for use. This quick, easy condiment is delicious in seafood soups, on steamed vegetables, or as an appetizer spread thinly onto small toasts. Makes approximately 1½ cups.

(Recipe created by Chef Gary Jenanyan.)

Garlic and Herb Dressing

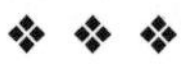

¼ cup Spectrum Essentials Flax Oil
¼ cup Spectrum Naturals Olive Oil
¼ cup + 1 tablespoon reduced-sodium soy sauce
3 tablespoons Spectrum Naturals Red Wine Vinegar
1 tablespoon mirin, white wine, or sherry (mirin is a rice vinegar that can be substituted for white wine)
¼ cup unsweetened ketchup
1 teaspoon lemon juice
¾ teaspoon vegetarian Worchestershire *sauce*
1 tablespoon crushed garlic (in the jar)
1 teaspoon Italian *herb seasoning*
1 teaspoon maple syrup

Blend together all the ingredients. For a thinner dressing, add more mirin. For a slightly spicier flavor, add a dash or two of hot sauce. Serve on salads and steamed vegetables such as broccoli and kale.

Honey Miso Sauce

❖ ❖ ❖

½ cup miso, red or yellow, or a combination
1 tablespoon Spectrum Naturals Toasted Sesame Oil
⅓ cup water
1½ tablespoons honey
1 teaspoon ginger, freshly grated (optional)
2 teaspoons Spectrum Naturals Brown Rice Vinegar
1 or 2 jalapeño or serrano chilies, seeded and pureed with a little water (optional)
salt and fresh-ground pepper to taste
cayenne pepper to taste (optional)
soy sauce to taste (optional)

Whisk miso, sesame oil, and water together until smooth. Mix in honey, ginger, and vinegar; add pureed chilies and salt and pepper to taste. For more heat, add up to ¼ teaspoon cayenne. If you are using a mild yellow miso, you may want to add a splash of soy sauce.

(Recipe adapted from *Field of Greens*, by Annie Somerville.)

Honey Sherry Dressing

❖ ❖ ❖

¾ cup oil
¼ cup wine vinegar
⅓ cup honey
1 teaspoon dry mustard
½ teaspoon paprika
½ teaspoon celery seed
1 clove garlic
1 cup sherry

Combine all ingredients in a jar or bowl. Shake or beat until well blended. Store, covered, in the refrigerator until needed, then shake or beat again before using. Garlic may be removed once its flavor has permeated the dressing. Excellent on fruits. Yield: about 1½–2 cups.

(Indian Summer, Inc.)

Make-Your-Own Salsa

❖ ❖ ❖

½ cup chopped red onion
¼ cup chopped green pepper
1 clove garlic, minced
1 tablespoon light olive oil
3 cups chopped very ripe fresh tomatoes
½ teaspoon oregano
3 tablespoons canned jalapeño peppers
2½ tablespoons Nakano Natural Rice Vinegar
2 tablespoons chopped fresh cilantro
¾ teaspoon salt
pepper as desired

Microwave onion, green pepper, garlic, and oil 1 minute on high, covered. Add tomatoes and oregano; microwave 2 minutes on high. Stir in remaining ingredients. Refrigerate an hour or overnight to blend flavor. Keeps for a week or freezes well. Makes about 3 cups sauce for 8–10 servings.

Nonfat Yogurt Cheese

❖ ❖ ❖

1 quart nonfat yogurt
4 tablespoons powdered sugar
2 teaspoons vanilla extract
1 tablespoon apple cider vinegar

Combine all above ingredients in a bowl. Whisk together until runny. Place strainer in a container that will hold it upright and also collect the liquid from the yogurt. Line strainer with double layer of cheesecloth. Pour in yogurt mixture. Leave overnight in refrigerator. Liquid will strain through. Remove from cheesecloth and store in refrigerator until ready to serve. A spread for bagels or toast. Makes about 1¼ cups of yogurt cheese. Serves 8.

(Chef Michel Stroot of the Golden Door Spa.)

New-Wave Italian Meat Sauce

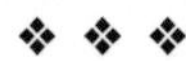

3 links (½ pound) mild Italian sausages
½ pound lean ground beef
2 tablespoons olive oil
½ cup chopped yellow onions
3 cloves garlic, minced
1 cup thickly sliced fresh mushrooms
1 (28-ounce) can crushed tomatoes in puree
¼ cup Nakano Italian Seasoned Red Wine Vinegar
¼ teaspoon pepper
¼ cup water
½ teaspoon salt (or as needed)
¼ teaspoon minced parsley

Remove sausage meat from casing. In large saucepan, brown sausage with ground beef using oil as needed. Add onion, garlic, and mushrooms and cook about 5 minutes with remaining oil. Stir in tomatoes, vinegar, and pepper. Simmer for 10 minutes. Add water and salt as desired. Stir in parsley. Makes 1 quart; 6 servings of ⅔ cup each. Serve over your favorite pasta, or bread as you would "Sloppy Joes."

Silken Tofu Tartare Sauce

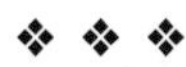

10 ounces silken soft tofu
¼ apple cider vinegar
1 tablespoon shallots, coarsely chopped
1 tablespoon Dijon mustard
2 teaspoons prepared horseradish, creamed
1 teaspoon finely ground black pepper
½ cup (Kosher) dill pickle, coarsely chopped
1 tablespoon capers
½ cup fresh parsley, coarsely chopped
2 teaspoons fresh tarragon, coarsely chopped
2 teaspoons fresh dill weed, or 1 teaspoon dried dill weed

In a blender, combine soft tofu, vinegar, shallots, Dijon mustard, horseradish, and black pepper and process until smooth. Add Kosher pickle, capers, parsley, tarragon, and dill to the blender. "Pulse" 5 to 6 times to keep the sauce "chunky." Makes about 2½ cups or forty 1-tablespoon servings. Serves 40.

(Chef Michel Stroot of the Golden Door Spa.)

Sweet and Sour Honey-Mustard Dipping Sauce

❖ ❖ ❖

4 teaspoons Dijon-style mustard
4 tablespoons Spectrum Naturals Seasoned Organic Brown Rice Vinegar
5 tablespoons honey
½ teaspoon salt
3 tablespoons water
2 tablespons Spectrum Naturals Pure Pressed Canola Oil (*or* Spectrum Naturals Super Canola Oil)
1 tablespoon garlic, finely minced
1 teaspoon arrowroot dissolved in 2 teaspoons water

Whisk together mustard, vinegar, honey, salt, and water in stainless steel or glass bowl. Reserve. Heat canola oil in skillet over medium heat. Add garlic, reduce heat, and stir constantly for 15 seconds. Do not burn. Add mustard mixture and simmer for 30 seconds. Add arrowroot and cook another 30 seconds, stirring constantly. Remove from heat and allow sauce to reach room temperature. This highly flavored sauce may be made several days in advance and gently reheated before serving. Excellent with cold vegetables, prepared tofu, or fish. Makes ¾ cup.

(Recipe created by Chef Gary Jenanyan.)

Quick Two-Tomato Sauce with Black Olives

2 tablespoons Spectrum Naturals Pure Pressed Canola Oil (*or* Spectrum Naturals Super Canola Oil)
1 medium yellow onion, minced
4 cloves garlic, minced
4 cups canned diced tomatoes or ripe garden tomatoes, peeled, seeded, and diced
⅓ cup dried tomatoes, chopped
½ cup black Niçoise *olives or black olives, pitted*
3 tablespoons fresh parsley, chopped
3 tablespoons fresh basil, chopped
2 tablespoons Spectrum Naturals Organic Red Wine Vinegar
3 tablespoons Spectrum Naturals Pressed Extra Virgin Olive Oil (*or* Certified Organic Extra Virgin, Imported Extra Virgin, *or* California Extra Virgin Olive Oil)
salt and fresh-ground pepper to taste

Warm canola oil in a 2- or 3-quart saucepan over medium heat. Add onions and sauté for 5 minutes. Add garlic and diced and dried tomatoes. Simmer for 15 minutes. Add olives and continue to simmer until all of the juice from the tomatoes has evaporated. Stir in parsley and basil. Simmer for 5 more minutes. Stir in vinegar and olive oil. Simmer for 5 more minutes, stirring often. Season with salt and fresh-ground pepper. Delicious with pasta, as an accompaniment to grilled or steamed fish, or simply spread cold on toast rounds as an appetizer. Makes approximately 2½ cups.

(Recipe created by Chef Gary Jenanyan.)

Vinaigrette Sauce for Vegetables

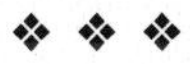

½ cup wine vinegar
1 cup olive oil
2 tablespoons red table wine
2 tablespoons chopped parsley
1½ teaspoons salt

Combine all ingredients in a covered jar and shake well. Serve on hot or cold cooked vegetables. Good on kidney beans or garbanzos. Yield: About 1½ cups.

(Indian Summer, Inc.)

Wine Butter Sauce for Fish

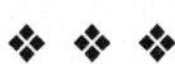

2 tablespoons chopped green onion
¼ teaspoon curry powder
½ cup butter
2 tablespoons wine vinegar
¼ cup white wine
2 tablespoons finely chopped parsley

Cook onion with curry powder gently in butter 3 or 4 minutes. Add remaining ingredients and heat gently. Spoon over cooked sole, salmon, lobster, or other fish. Yield: About ⅔ cup.

(Indian Summer, Inc.)

Pasta

Vegetables, fruits, and some grains make up a big part of the Mediterranean diet. Pasta with vinegar, garlic, onions, and olive oil is a healthy meal.

What is it about pasta that makes it such a diet-friendly choice? Simple: It's low in fat and sodium and has just about 200 calories per 2-ounce serving (about 1 cup).

Pasta's also a good source of fiber, so it's extra-filling. And if you switch to whole wheat pasta, which contains more bulk, you'll feel even more satisfied. In addition, fiber can stabilize blood sugar levels, say nutritionists, which keeps your appetite at bay.

Pasta is also high in nutrition, containing calcium, iron, niacin, magnesium, and protein. What more could a health-conscious pasta lover want?

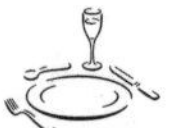

Dill Tomato Pasta Salad
Orzo and Vegetable Salad
Gnocchi Pasta Shells with Toasted Garlic and Pancetta
Pasta Primavera Salad
Piquant Prawns with Tomato and Linguini
Spinach Salad with Italian Sausage Pompeian
Tart and Spicy Thai Noodles
Venetian Pasta Salad

Dill Tomato Pasta Salad

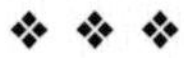

Full of flavor yet light on the fat, you'll make this pasta salad over and over—it's so easy!

1 (14½-ounce) can diced tomatoes in juice
¼ cup Nakano White Wine Vinegar
¼ cup salad oil or olive oil
½ teaspoon each sugar, salt, and pepper
½ teaspoon dill weed
1 small clove garlic, minced
8 ounces rotini, cooked and drained
½ cup each sliced celery, cucumber, and green onion
½ cup julienned carrots
2 tablespoons chopped parsley

In a large salad bowl, combine tomatoes, vinegar, oil, sugar, salt, pepper, dill, and garlic; stir. Add remaining ingredients; toss to combine. Stir before serving. Serves 6–8.

Orzo and Vegetable Salad

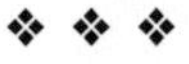

1 cup orzo (rice-shaped pasta)
¼ cup Heinz Apple Cider Vinegar
¼ cup vegetable oil
1 teaspoon Dijon-style mustard
½ teaspoon dried basil leaves
¼ teaspoon salt
⅛ teaspoon pepper
1 cup frozen green peas, thawed
4 green onions, sliced
½ cup chopped red bell pepper
lettuce cups
tomato wedges

Cook orzo according to package directions; cool. Combine vinegar and next 5 ingredients in jar. Cover and shake vigorously. Chill to blend flavors. Combine orzo, peas, onions, and bell pepper in large bowl. Pour dressing over and toss. Cover, and chill several hours or overnight. Serve in lettuce cups; garnish with tomato. Makes 4 servings (about 5 cups).

Gnocchi Pasta Shells with Toasted Garlic and Pancetta

❖ ❖ ❖

1 cup Spectrum Naturals Super Canola Oil
1 head garlic cloves, peeled
½ cup Spectrum Naturals Extra Virgin Olive Oil
2 cups organic diced tomatoes
4 ounces pancetta bacon, cut into cubes and rendered
2 tablespoons Spectrum Naturals Organic Balsamic Vinegar
1 teaspoon red chili flakes (optional)
8 ounces gnocchi pasta shells
6 tablespoons fresh basil, chopped
6 tablespoons fresh parsley, chopped
salt and fresh ground pepper to taste

Bring 6 quarts of water to a boil with a tablespoon of salt. While water is boiling, heat canola oil in a saucepan. Add the garlic cloves and toast them in the hot oil until golden brown, about 3 or 4 minutes, stirring constantly. Remove garlic with a slotted spoon to paper towels and set aside. Reserve the now garlic-flavored canola oil for another use. Warm olive oil in a large sauté pan. Add the tomatoes, toasted garlic, and rendered pancetta. Add balsamic vinegar and continue to cook over low heat. Stir in the optional chili flakes. Remove from the heat and reserve while the pasta cooks. Cook the pasta, drain, and add to the sauté pan. Add the basil and parsley, and mix well. Check the seasoning and serve immediately.

(Recipe created by Chef Gary Jenanyan.)

Pasta Primavera Salad

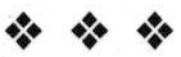

8 ounces twisted noodles or tortellini
½ cup light french dressing (see below)
1 cup fresh asparagus
1 cup small broccoli flowerets
1 cup frozen peas, thawed
½ cup sweet red pepper strips
½ cup celery
¼ cup chopped red onion
1 clove garlic, minced
black pepper, to taste
4 ounces reduced-fat Monterey Jack cheese, cubed
¼ cup grated Parmesan cheese

Cook noodles or tortellini as directed; drain and rinse in cold water. Place in serving bowl, toss with dressing, and chill.

Combine all vegetables and garlic in a glass casserole dish. Microwave, covered, on high power for 3–4 minutes or until cooked tender-crisp; cool. Toss vegetables with noodles. Season with black pepper, if desired. Chill at least ½ hour. Stir in both cheeses. Best served same day. Serves 4.

Light French Dressing

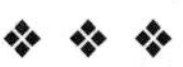

½ cup Nakano Seasoned Apple Cider *or* Red Wine Vinegar
¼ cup light olive oil
½ teaspoon Dijon mustard
¼ teaspoon fine herbs
¼ teaspoon celery seed
pinch of black pepper
1 clove garlic, sliced

Combine all ingredients except garlic and blend. Pour into jar; add garlic. Let stand at room temperature at least ½ hour. Shake well before using. Keeps well. Makes ¾ cup dressing.

Piquant Prawns with Tomato and Linguine

❖ ❖ ❖

½ *cup* Spectrum Naturals Organic Extra Virgin Olive Oil
6 cloves garlic, peeled and minced
3 *tablespoons* Spectrum Naturals Organic Red Wine Vinegar
1 (14.5-ounce) can, diced tomatoes
1 teaspoon red chili flakes (optional)
1 pound large prawns, shelled and deveined
8 ounces linguine
5 tablespoons fresh basil, chopped
5 tablespoons fresh parsley, chopped
salt and fresh-ground pepper to taste

For pasta, boil 6 quarts of water with a tablespoon of salt. Meanwhile, gently warm olive oil in a large sauté pan. Add garlic and begin to cook. Add vinegar and tomatoes, and continue to cook over low heat. Stir in the chili flakes. Add prawns and simmer until just cooked through, turning often, about 5 minutes. Remove from heat, reserve while pasta cooks. Drain pasta and toss together with prawns. Add basil, parsley, salt, and pepper. Check the seasoning and serve immediately.

(Recipe created by Chef Gary Jenanyan.)

Spinach Salad with Italian Sausage Pompeian

❖ ❖ ❖

4 cups packed stemmed spinach, torn into bite-sized pieces
1 *teaspoon* Pompeian Extra Virgin Olive Oil
4 sweet turkey meat Italian sausages
3 green onions, sliced
3 tablespoons Pompeian Red Wine Vinegar
1 *tablespoon* Pompeian Extra Virgin Olive Oil
1 teaspoon Dijon mustard
salt and fresh ground pepper to taste

Place spinach in a large bowl. Heat 1 teaspoon olive oil in a large skillet over medium heat. Add sausages and cook until browned and cooked through. Remove pan from heat and leave drippings in the pan. Drain sausages on paper towel then slice ½-inch thick. Heat drippings over medium heat. Add green onions and stir 1 minute. Add vinegar and bring to a boil, scraping up any browned bits. Mix in 1 tablespoon of olive oil and mustard. Add sausage and toss to coat. Season with salt and pepper. Pour over spinach and toss. Serves 2.

Tart and Spicy Thai Noodles

❖ ❖ ❖

- 3 *tablespoons* Spectrum World Cuisine Thai Seasoning Oil
- 3 *tablespoons* Spectrum Naturals Organic Unrefined Toasted Sesame Oil
- 4 *tablespoons tamari soy sauce*
- 3 *tablespoons* Spectrum Naturals Organic White Wine Vinegar
- 2 *tablespoons honey*
- 12 *ounces fresh Chinese-style thin egg noodles*
- *salt and fresh ground pepper to taste*
- 4 *scallions, chopped*
- 3 *tablespoons cilantro, chopped*
- 3 *tablespoons peanuts, coarsely chopped*

Boil 6 quarts of lightly salted water. Meanwhile, whisk together Thai oil, sesame oil, soy sauce, vinegar, and honey in a large bowl. Cook noodles in salted water, approximately 3 minutes. Drain thoroughly and transfer to the bowl with seasonings; toss well. Season with salt and pepper; mix in scallions and cilantro. Let sit for 5 minutes to absorb the seasonings. Toss well and sprinkle with peanuts. Serve warm or cold.

(Recipe created by Chef Gary Jenanyan.)

Venetian Pasta Salad

❖ ❖ ❖

8 ounces thin spaghetti, uncooked
½ cup julienned red bell pepper
½ cup julienned green bell pepper
4 ounces Swiss cheese, cut into ½-inch cubes
⅓ cup coarsely chopped pitted calamata or ripe olives
*¼ cup chopped walnuts, toasted**
¼ cup grated Parmesan cheese
¼ cup packed fresh basil leaves, chopped
1 tablespoon chopped flat leaf parsley
3 tablespoons olive oil
2 tablespoons Nakano Seasoned Red Wine Vinegar—Italian Herb
1 clove garlic, minced
¼ teaspoon salt
¼ teaspoon sugar
freshly ground black pepper

Break spaghetti in half; cook according to package directions. Drain; rinse with cold water. Drain well; transfer to a large bowl. Add bell peppers, Swiss cheese, olives, walnuts, Parmesan cheese, basil, and parsley; mix well. In a small bowl whisk together the olive oil, vinegar, garlic, salt, and sugar; pour over spaghetti mixture. Combine all ingredients; cover and chill. Serve chilled or at room temperature with pepper. Serves 4.

*To toast walnuts, arrange on a small baking sheet and bake in a 350° oven 6–8 minutes or until golden brown and fragrant.

Vegetables/Vegetarian

Vegetables are the key to staying healthy and paring off pounds. "Vegetables fill you up because they're high in fiber, which helps keep you from overeating," says Jay Kenney, Ph.D., R.D., of the Pritikin Longevity Center in Santa Monica, California. "And ounce for ounce, they're lower in calories than other foods."

Vegetables are also an excellent source of complex carbohydrates. Complex carbs raise the brain's levels of serotonin, a chemical that works to diminish hunger.

Another big benefit: Vegetables are chock-full of the antioxidant vitamins C, E, and beta-carotene (which converts into vitamin A). These vitamins trap the free-radical molecules that cause normal cells to become cancerous, says Connie Mobley, Ph.D., R.D., of the University of Texas Health Sciences Center in San Antonio. According to the American Cancer Society, studies show that a diet high in vegetables can lower cancer risk.

In our recipes you can pair vegetables with apple cider, red wine, and herbal vinegars, then toss in garlic, onions, and olive oil. The result? You've got a powerhouse of health-enhancing food and mouthwatering dishes to savor.

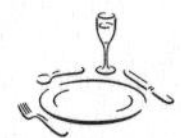

Asparagus with Leeks and Capers
Baked Sweet Potatoes with Plantain and Citrus Chutney
Caponata
Garden Vegetable Potpourri
Italian-Style Marinated Tomatoes
Greek Pita Pizza
Marinated Green Vegetables
Marinated Mushrooms and Vegetables with Blueberry Vinegar
Simmered Lentils with Winter Vegetables
Steamed Artichokes with Yogurt and Buttermilk Dressing
Swedish Red Cabbage
White Bean and Fennel Sauté

Asparagus with Leeks And Capers

❖ ❖ ❖

½ pound fresh asparagus, stalks trimmed
1 leek, thinly sliced (white and light green part only)
1 small red bell pepper, cut into short, thin strips
⅓ cup extra virgin olive oil
3 tablespoons Nakano Seasoned Rice Vinegar with Basil & Oregano *or* Seasoned Red Wine Vinegar
1 tablespoon chopped fresh thyme or ½ teaspoon dried thyme leaves
½ teaspoon salt
¼ teaspoon fresh ground black pepper
8 Boston or 12 bib lettuce leaves
½ cup garlic croutons
2 tablespoons bottled capers, drained
1 ounce Parmesan cheese

Bring a large pot of water to a boil. Add asparagus, leek, and bell pepper. Return to a boil; simmer uncovered 1 minute. Drain and immediately transfer vegetables to a bowl of ice water to stop the cooking and set the color. Let stand 5 minutes; drain well and transfer to a shallow dish. Combine oil, vinegar, thyme, salt, and pepper; mix well. Pour evenly over vegetables; cover and chill at least 2 hours or up to 24 hours before serving. Arrange lettuce leaves on four serving plates; top attractively with vegetables. Drizzle remaining dressing from dish evenly over salads; top with croutons and capers. Using a rotary blade vegetable peeler, shave cheese over salads. Serves 4.

Baked Sweet Potaotes with Plantain and Citrus Chutney

❖ ❖ ❖

4 medium sweet potatoes, washed and pierced with a fork
2 tablespoons peanut or vegetable oil
1 ripe plantain, peeled, cut into ½-inch cubes
2 teaspoons water
2 tablespoons diced red onion
2 tablespoons Nakano Natural Rice Vinegar
2 tablespoons orange juice
1 tablespoon lime juice
2 tablespoons brown sugar
1 teaspoon grated lime zest
dash of nutmeg
dash of ground cloves
1 tablespoon butter
1 large naval orange, peeled, separated into sections, sections halved

Preheat oven to 425°. Place potatoes on a cookie sheet lined with foil and bake until cooked through, 40–45 minutes. Meanwhile, heat oil in a nonstick skillet over medium heat. Add plantain, cover, and cook 3–4 minutes or until golden brown, stirring once. Add water, cover, and cook an additional 2 minutes or until liquid is absorbed. Add onion, cook 1 minute. Combine vinegar, orange and lime juices, brown sugar, zest, nutmeg, and cloves, mixing until sugar dissolves. Add to the pan; simmer over medium-high heat until sauce thickens. Stir in butter and orange sections; heat through. When potatoes are finished baking, split them open and top with orange mixture. Serves 4.

Caponata
(Sicilian Eggplant Appetizer)

❖ ❖ ❖

2½ pounds eggplant
salt
6–8 stalks of celery (11 to 12 ounces, green parts only)
canola oil and olive oil
1 onion, chopped
3 or 4 cloves garlic, chopped fine
2¼ cups tomato sauce or 3 large tomatoes, peeled, seeded, and diced
½ cup parsley, chopped
8 ounces green olives, pitted and halved
3 ounces small capers, drained and rinsed
freshly ground black pepper to taste
1 cup red wine vinegar
2 tablespoons sugar

Peel or partially peel the eggplant and cut into ¾-inch cubes. Rinse and sprinkle with salt and drain in a colander while slicing celery into ½-inch pieces. Parboil celery for 5 minutes. Drain and set aside. In a large skillet, pour canola oil and olive oil (canola oil has a higher smoking point than olive oil, making it better for frying) about a half-inch deep over medium heat. After drying the eggplant, add it to hot oil mixture and brown all sides. Remove with slotted spoon and drain on paper towels and cover and pat with more paper towels. In another skillet, sauté onion and garlic in olive oil Cook slowly, until the onions are golden (10 or 12 minutes). Do not brown. Add tomato sauce, parsley, olives, capers, and salt and pepper to taste. Stir together and bring to a boil. Stir in the red wine vinegar and sugar. Reduce heat and simmer for 15 minutes. Remove from heat and spoon in the eggplant, stirring to mix thoroughly. Taste to adjust seasoning. Remove as much liquid as possible and serve or cool for later service. Caponata will last for a week when refrigerated. It is usually served cold. Serves 8–10.

Garden Vegetable Potpourri

❖ ❖ ❖

1 quart prepared vegetables:
cauliflower flowerets; peeled baby carrots or slices; celery, cut into 1-inch pieces
red onion wedges
zucchini wedges or slices
sweet red pepper squares
green pepper squares
1 teaspoon whole peppercorns
½ teaspoon fine herbs
1 clove garlic, diced
1 stalk basil (optional)
1½ cups (approx.) Seasoned Nakano Apple Cider Vinegar

In a large saucepan, parboil cauliflower, carrots, and celery 5 minutes. Remove from heat and add onion, zucchini, red and green pepper; drain immediately, saving some liquid. Rinse vegetables in cold water. In a quart jar, place peppercorns, herbs, and garlic. Pour in 2 tablespoons hot vegetable cooking water; let stand a few minutes. Pack cool vegetables in jar, adding basil to center. Push vegetables down tightly to fill jar. Top off with vinegar; cover and shake. Refrigerate overnight. Keeps well for several weeks. Makes 1 quart.

Italian-Style Marinated Tomatoes

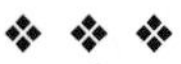

3 large tomatoes, sliced
salt and pepper
¼ cup Nakano Red Wine Vinegar
3 tablespoons chopped fresh basil (or 1 teaspoon dried basil, crushed)
2 tablespoons olive oil
2 teaspoons brown sugar
1 small clove garlic, minced
shredded Parmesan cheese
whole basil leaves

Arrange tomatoes on a serving platter or in a large shallow bowl. Sprinkle lightly with salt and pepper. Combine remaining ingredients except cheese; stir to dissolve sugar. Let stand 10 minutes. Drizzle over tomatoes; marinate just 5 minutes. Sprinkle tomatoes with cheese and garnish with whole basil leaves. Serve with crusty Italian bread and slices of fresh mozzarella, if desired. Makes 4 appetizer servings.

Greek Pita Pizza

❖ ❖ ❖

6 pita bread rounds (thick, Greek style are best)
2 tablespoons Spectrum Naturals Mediterranean Spread
1-ounce bag organic spinach leaves
½ red onion, thinly sliced
1 medium tomato, diced
1 large clove garlic, finely minced
1 medium yellow bell pepper, finely chopped
8 Kalamata or Gaeta Olives, pitted and chopped
6 pepperoncini peppers, cut in half lengthwise
6 ounces feta cheese, crumbled
2 tablespoons Spectrum Naturals Olive Oil
1 tablespoon Spectrum Naturals Red Wine Vinegar
1 tablespoon freshly squeezed lemon juice
1 teaspoon dried oregano
salt and pepper to taste

Preheat the oven to 350°. Arrange the pita rounds on two nonstick cookie sheets. Spread the Mediterranean Spread evenly over the pita breads, using a butter knife or a rubber spatula. Bake in the preheated oven 5 minutes. Transfer the pita rounds to a large serving platter. Meanwhile, in a large bowl, combine the spinach leaves, onion, tomato, garlic, bell pepper, olives, pepperoncini, and feta cheese. Toss gently to combine. In a separate bowl combine the olive oil, vinegar, lemon juice, oregano, salt (add only a little salt, the feta and olives are salty) and pepper to taste. Whisk to combine. Pour this dressing over the tossed spinach mixture; toss well to combine. Taste for seasonings. Divide the salad mixture evenly over the pita rounds. Serve immediately.

(Recipe created by Claire Criscullo.)

Marinated Green Vegetables

1 pound broccoli florets
1 pound asparagus, fresh spears
1 pound zucchini, fresh and firm
½ cup extra virgin olive oil
1 large yellow onion, sliced thin
4 garlic cloves, finely chopped
2 fresh basil leaves, chopped into ¼-inch strips
2 fresh sage leaves, chopped into ¼-inch strips
a pinch of salt
1 cup red wine vinegar

Blanch broccoli in salted boiling water for 2 minutes. Remove and set aside. Blanch asparagus spears in same water for 1 minute or less. Set aside. Wash zucchini in cold water and cut into ¼-inch strips about 3 inches long. Heat 2 tablespoons of the olive oil in a skillet and sauté the zucchini strips over high heat until a little color is attained. Do not cook until limp. Use as little oil as possible. Remove while still al dente (firm to the bite). Set aside. In the same skillet, add more oil if needed and sauté the sliced onion until brown. Add the garlic, chopped basil, chopped sage, and pinch of salt. Before the garlic turns brown, add the vinegar, bring to a boil, and then reduce until there is just a little liquid left in the pan. Combine the set-aside green vegetables and pour the onion, garlic, and vinegar mixture over them. Toss to flavor all pieces. Serve at room temperature or save for later service. Serves 8 to 10.

(Recipe by Chef Salvatore J. Campagna.)

Marinated Mushrooms and Vegetables with Blueberry Vinegar

❖ ❖ ❖

¾ cup olive oil
½ cup of water
⅓ cup blueberry vinegar
1 tablespoon salt
2 cups small fresh caulifIowerets
1 pound medium fresh mushrooms, rinsed and halved
½ of a 7.5-ounces jar roasted sweet red peppers, drained and cut in strips
1 medium onion, minced
½ teaspoon pepper
3 medium green peppers, seeded and cut in 1-inch strips
1 tablespoon dried basil

Mix the dressing and marinate the veggies overnight. Very pretty addition to a buffet table or picnic.

(Courtesy of Valley View Blueberries.)

Simmered Lentils with Winter Vegetables

❖ ❖ ❖

1 pound brown lentils
1 carrot, peeled and diced
2 stalks celery, diced
salt and fresh ground pepper to taste
1 medium red onion, finely diced
4 tablespoons Mediterranean *or* Only Olive Spectrum Spread
1 tablespoon or more Spectrum Naturals Organic Red Wine Vinegar
½ cup Italian parsley, finely chopped

Place the lentils in a large casserole dish and cover with cold water. Bring to a simmer over medium heat. Simmer the lentils gently for about 20 minutes or until they are no longer starchy-raw inside. Add the carrots and continue to cook another 10 minutes. Season with salt and pepper. Stir in the celery and onions. Continue to cook until the lentils are completely done, about 10 more minutes, adding more water as necessary. Stir in the Spectrum Spread to enrich the flavor. Stir in the vinegar. Check seasonings. Stir in the parsley. Serve. Makes 6–8 servings.

Steamed Artichokes with Yogurt And Buttermilk Dressing

½ cup low-fat buttermilk
⅓ cup low-fat plain yogurt
2 tablespoons Nakano Seasoned Rice Vinegar with Basil & Oregano *or* Nakano Seasoned Rice Vinegar with Red Pepper
2 tablespoons lite or regular mayonnaise
2 tablespoons chopped fresh or 2 teaspoons dried basil
1 clove garlic, minced (optional)
2 teaspoons sugar
1 teaspoon Dijon-style mustard
⅛ teaspoon salt
⅛ teaspoon oregano
⅛ teaspoon freshly ground black pepper, or to taste
4 fresh artichokes (about 6 ounces each), stems and leaves trimmed

Combine all ingredients except artichokes in a small bowl; mix well. Cover and refrigerate at least 1 hour. Steam artichokes 25–35 minutes or until leaves pull out easily. Serve hot or cold with dressing. Serves 4.

Swedish Red Cabbage

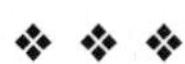

1 package (8 ounces or 1 quart) prepared shredded red cabbage
½ cup water
⅓ cup Nakano Seasoned Red Wine Vinegar
2 tablespoons diced red onion
1 tablespoon canola oil
pinch ground allspice
pinch black pepper
2 cups chopped peeled apples
1 tablespoon raspberry jelly

In a glass casserole dish, combine all ingredients except apples and jelly. Microwave, covered, on high power for 10 minutes; stir. Microwave on medium power for 10 minutes. Stir in apples and jelly; microwave 5 more minutes on medium. Serve hot or cold. Great side dish with turkey, pork, or pot roast. Keeps well for 3–4 days. Serves 8.

White Bean and Fennel Sauté

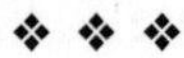

1 large fennel bulb, about 10 ounces
1 tablespoon olive oil
1 small onion, thinly sliced
2 cloves garlic, minced
½ cup diced yellow bell pepper
3 tablespoons Nakano Seasoned Rice Vinegar with Roasted Garlic *or* Nakano Seasoned Rice Vinegar—Original
¼ teaspoon salt, or to taste
⅛ teaspoon freshly ground black pepper
1 (10 ounce) can cannellini beans, rinsed and drained

Trim off stems of fennel bulb. If desired, chop enough feathery fennel fronds to measure 2 tablespoons; set aside. Thinly slice fennel bulb. In a medium skillet, heat olive oil over medium-high heat. Add sliced fennel, onion, and garlic; cook until soft and fragrant, about 4 minutes, stirring occasionally. Add bell pepper, vinegar, salt, and pepper; mix well and cook 1 minute. Add beans; heat through. Serve warm, at room temperature, or chilled. Serves 4.

Seafood

Fish contains the omega-3 fatty acids (which are found in salmon, swordfish, and tuna), potassium, and only a small amount of sodium. And it's these ingredients that help you have lower blood pressure and cholesterol levels. That means you'll be less prone to heart attacks and strokes.

What's more, when you include heart-healthy vinegar, garlic, onions, and olive oil with fish, as in our tantalizing fish recipes, you'll be on track to keeping a healthy heart.

Classic Seviche
Crab Cakes With Nakano Vinegar Mayonnaise
Grilled Tuna with Fresh Tomato,
Cucumber, and Dill Relish
Jerk Swordfish with Fresh Pineapple Salsa
Sesame Fish with Sautéed Spinach
Roast Salmon with Balsamic Glaze
Simple Salmon
Stir-Fry Shrimp and Rice
Tapa-Style Mussels

Classic Seviche

1 pound bay scallops or firm white fish fillets, cut into 1-inch cubes
*1/4 cup fresh lime juice**
1/2 cup Nakano Seasoned Rice Vinegar with Red Pepper *or* Nakano Seasoned Rice Vinegar—Original
3/4 cup diced red and/or green bell pepper
1/3 cup chopped red onion
1 clove garlic, minced
1/2 teaspoon hot pepper sauce, or 1 jalapeño pepper, minced
assorted crackers, melba toast, or large corn tortilla chips

Place scallops in a shallow 1½-quart casserole dish. Pour lime juice over scallops; mix well and press into an even layer. In a small bowl, combine remaining ingredients; pour over scallops. Cover and refrigerate at least 24 hours or until scallops are opaque. Transfer mixture with a slotted spoon to a serving bowl. Discard marinade. Serve with crackers. Serves 5.

*Fresh lime juice and vinegar "cook" the scallops as they marinate overnight.

Crab Cakes with Nakano Vinegar Mayonnaise

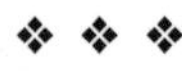

1/2 pound lump crab meat or 2 (6-ounce) cans crab meat, rinsed, drained
1 egg
1 green onion, chopped
1/2 teaspoon seasoned salt
1/8 teaspoon cayenne pepper
2½ tablespoons plus 1/4 cup dry bread crumbs
1 tablespoon vegetable oil
3/4 cup lite or regular mayonnaise
3 tablespoons Nakano Seasoned Rice Vinegar with Red Pepper *or* Nakano Seasoned Rice Vinegar—Original
2 teaspoons Dijon-style mustard

Pick over crab meat, discarding any bits of shell. In a medium bowl, combine crab meat, egg, green onion, salt, and cayenne pepper. Add

2½ tablespoons bread crumbs. Mix well; shape into four patties about 3 inches wide and ½-inch thick. (Note: At this point, crab cakes may be covered and refrigerated up to 4 hours before cooking.) Place remaining ¼ cup bread crumbs on a shallow plate. Dip crab cakes in bread crumbs, patting to coat lightly. Heat oil in a large nonstick skillet over medium heat. Add crab cakes; cook about 4 minutes per side or until golden brown. Meanwhile, combine mayonnaise, vinegar, and mustard; mix well. Serve crab cakes with mayonnaise. Serves 4.

Grilled Tuna with Fresh Tomato, Cucumber, and Dill Relish

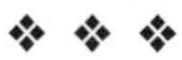

4 tablespoons Nakano Seasoned Rice Vinegar with Basil & Oregano *or* Nakano Seasoned Rice Vinegar with Roasted Garlic
¼ cup plus 1 tablespoon olive oil
¾ teaspoon oregano
¼ teaspoon plus ⅛ teaspoon salt
¼ teaspoon freshly ground black pepper
4 (6 to 8 ounces) fresh tuna steaks, cut ¾-inch thick
1 cup seeded, diced ripe tomato
⅔ cup peeled, seeded, diced cucumber
1½ teaspoons chopped fresh dill

Combine 2 tablespoons vinegar, ¼ cup olive oil, oregano, ¼ teaspoon salt, and ⅛ teaspoon pepper; mix well. Place tuna in a shallow dish or resealable plastic bag and top with vinegar mixture, turning fish to coat both sides. Cover dish or close bag securely; refrigerate at least 15 minutes or up to 2 hours before grilling. Meanwhile, in a small bowl, combine tomato, cucumber, dill, and remaining 2 tablespoons vinegar, 1 tablespoon olive oil, ⅛ teaspoon each salt and pepper; mix well. Relish may be chilled or served at room temperature. Drain fish, discarding marinade. Place on grill over medium-hot coals; grill 3 minutes per side (fish will be pink in center). Serve warm or at room temperature topped with relish. Serves 4.

Jerk Swordfish with Fresh Pineapple Salsa

Marinade

1 medium red onion, coarsely chopped
1 jalapeño pepper, seeded and minced or 2 teaspoons bottled minced jalapeño peppers
½ cup lite soy sauce
½ cup natural rice vinegar
¼ cup olive oil
¼ cup brown sugar
1½ teaspoons Caribbean jerk seasoning
1 teaspoon dried thyme
1 teaspoon cracked black pepper
½ teaspoon chopped fresh ginger
4 (6–8-ounces) fresh swordfish steaks, cut ¾-inch thick

Pineapple Salsa

2 cups diced fresh pineapple
½ cup chopped red onion
½ cup chopped fresh cilantro
2 tablespoons chopped fresh mint
2 tablespoons natural rice vinegar
¼ teaspoon cayenne pepper
salt to taste

For marinade, combine all ingredients except fish in a food processor. Process 10 seconds. Place fish in resealable plastic bag. Pour marinade over fish; close bag securely, turning to coat. Refrigerate at least 4 hours or overnight. For salsa, combine all ingredients in a medium bowl; refrigerate at least 1 hour or overnight. Drain fish, discarding marinade. Grill over medium-hot coals or broil 4–5 inches from heat source about 5 minutes per side or until fish is opaque. Serve with salsa. Serve warm or at room temperature with pineapple. Serves 4.

Sesame Fish with Sautéed Spinach

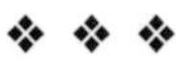

3 *tablespoons* Nakano Seasoned Rice Vinegar—Original *or* Nakano Seasoned Rice Vinegar with Red Pepper
2 *tablespoons lite or regular teriyaki sauce*
1 *tablespoon vegetable oil*
2 *teaspoons dark roasted sesame oil*
1 *teaspoon bottled or fresh minced ginger*
¼ *teaspoon crushed red pepper flakes*
4 *(4–5-ounces) skinless halibut, red snapper, or orange roughy fish fillets*
1 *(10-ounce) package washed spinach leaves, stems discarded*
2 *teaspoons sesame seeds, toasted (optional)*

Combine vinegar, teriyaki sauce, vegetable oil, sesame oil, ginger, and pepper flakes; mix well. Set aside half of mixture. Place fish on a shallow plate; drizzle remaining vinegar mixture evenly over fish. Turn fish to coat both sides. Let stand at room temperature 20 minutes. Place fish on rack of broiler pan or on grid over medium coals. Brush fish with any remaining marinade from dish. Broil fish 4–5 inches from heat source 5 minutes. Turn; continue to broil 4–5 minutes, or until fish is opaque. While fish is cooking, heat remaining vinegar mixture in a large deep skillet over medium-high heat. Add spinach; cover and simmer 1–2 minutes or until spinach is wilted. Transfer with tongs to four serving plates. Arrange fish over spinach; drizzle with any remaining vinegar mixture from skillet. Sprinkle with sesame seeds, if desired. Serves 4.

Roast Salmon with Balsamic Glaze

❖ ❖ ❖

5-pound whole salmon center, bone removed
1 tablespoon grated lemon rind
2 cloves garlic, finely chopped
2 tablespoons chopped fresh thyme
3 tablespoons olive oil
½ cup balsamic vinegar
½ cup red wine
1 teaspoon granulated sugar
¼ cup butter
lemon slices

Preheat oven to 350°. Place salmon in baking dish. Chop together lemon rind, garlic, and thyme. Brush oil over salmon and inside cavity. Rub herb mixture over. (Prepare up to 24 hours ahead of time.) Roast 40 minutes or until white juices appear on top. Meanwhile, combine balsamic vinegar, wine, and sugar in a skillet. Bring to boil and reduce until syrupy. Turn heat to low and whisk in butter. Remove skin from salmon. Serve with sauce and lemon slices. Serves 8–10.

(The Vinegar Institute.)

Simple Salmon
Marinate and Bake the Salmon in the Same Pan

6 filets, 6 ounces each
1 tomato, peeled, seeded, and diced
4 ounces yellow onion, sliced
2 ounces carrots, sliced
1 lemon, sliced into rounds
2 cloves garlic, sliced
8 ounces vegetable broth
2 ounces olive oil
2 ounces red wine vinegar
2 ounces dry red wine
2 bay leaves
3 fresh thyme sprigs
4 fresh tarragon leaves
salt and pepper to taste

Place the 6 salmon filets in an oven-proof glass pan. Add all the other ingredients. Marinate for 1 hour in the refrigerator. In the same glass pan, cover salmon loosely with a piece of foil and bake for 15 minutes at 350°. When salmon is done, remove to a service plate. Strain liquid from baking pan and reduce to less than a cup using a whisk. Adjust seasoning and pour over salmon. Serves 6.

(Recipe by Chef Salvatore J. Campagna.)

Stir-Fry Shrimp and Rice

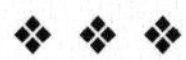

3 green onions, sliced
½ cup chopped green bell pepper
½ cup chopped red bell pepper
1 pound tiny cocktail shrimp
1 quart cooked long-grain rice, cold
1 (8-ounce) can pineapple chunks in juice
⅓ cup natural rice vinegar
3 tablespoon Oriental sesame oil
pinch pepper
¼ cup chopped fresh cilantro
½ cup sliced natural almonds

In a large nonstick skillet or wok, stir-fry onions with green and red pepper for a few minutes. Stir in shrimp and rice. Add pineapple with juice, vinegar, oil, and pepper. Heat thoroughly. Toss in cilantro. Garnish with almonds. Serve hot, or for salad, divide mixture into 4 small molds and chill 2 hours or overnight. Unmold salads onto lettuce leaves. Makes six (1-cup) servings.

Tapas-Style Mussels

❖ ❖ ❖

24 large live mussels, scrubbed
½ cup water
¼ cup finely chopped red bell pepper
¼ cup finely chopped yellow bell pepper
¼ cup finely chopped pitted calamata or ripe olives
2 tablespoons Nakano Seasoned Rice Vinegar with Basil & Oregano *or* Nakano Seasoned Rice Vinegar—Original
2 tablespoons extra virgin olive oil
1 clove garlic, minced

Combine mussels and water in a large deep skillet or Dutch oven. Cover; bring to a boil over high heat. Reduce heat to medium; continue to cook until mussels open, 4–5 minutes. Discard any mussels that do not open. Drain mussels; cool to room temperature. Meanwhile, combine remaining ingredients; mix well. Remove and discard one side of each mussel shell, leaving mussel in remaining shell. Arrange mussels on a serving platter. Spoon about 1 teaspoon vinegar mixture over each mussel. Serve at room temperature or chilled. Serves 8–12.

Tip: Most mussels are now farm-raised and contain very little sand and grit, but if the mussels are harvested from the ocean, soak them in cold water with a tablespoon of cornmeal and rinse them well before scrubbing.

Poultry

Protein helps you shed weight by decreasing your body's production of insulin. This is important because insulin locks fat in your fat cells, according to nutritionists.

You can keep insulin levels low by increasing your intake of protein-rich foods like skinless chicken and lean turkey meat.

Protein has just 4 calories per gram—about half the number of calories fat has. Says Columbus, Georgia, weight-loss specialist Jan McBaron, M.D., "Protein is digested slowly, so it helps curb your appetite." And protein-rich poultry is also rich in other nutrients.

And remember, season your food with spices such as garlic, pepper, and oregano. Lemon juice, vinegar, and hot sauce add zest without adding fat.

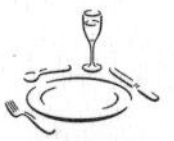

Chicken Bite Appetizers
Chicken Breasts with Blueberries
Crispy Hot and Tangy Thai Chicken
Grilled Marinated Chicken
Mediterranean Simmered Chicken
Polynesian Chicken
Seared Chicken Breast Stuffed with Spinach
Sesame Chicken Sautéed with Broccoli
Sweet and Sour Chicken
Tomato and Herb Chicken
Tangy Chicken and Herbs
Turkey Wraps

Chicken Bite Appetizers

❖ ❖ ❖

2 whole chicken breasts (boned and skinned)
paprika, salt, and pepper
1 tablespoon Pompeian Red Wine Vinegar
⅓ cup Pompeian Extra Virgin Olive Oil

Cut chicken into bite-sized pieces, sprinkle with paprika, salt, and pepper. Add vinegar and stir well to coat all the pieces. Marinate in refrigerator for at least 1 hour. Heat olive oil in skillet to 320°. Add chicken and sauté both sides until golden brown (about 3 minutes). Serve immediately on wooden toothpicks.

Chicken Breasts with Blueberries

❖ ❖ ❖

2 tablespoons butter or margarine
2 whole chicken breasts cut in half and skinned
⅓ cup peach or apricot jam
3 tablespoons Dijon mustard
⅓ cup blueberries (fresh, frozen, or dried)
½ cup blueberry vinegar

In a 10–12-inch frying pan over medium-high heat, melt butter and add chicken. Cook until brown then turn. Meanwhile, mix jam and mustard then spread over meaty side of breasts. Sprinkle with blueberries. Turn heat to medium-low and cook covered until done, about 15 minutes. With a slotted spoon, lift chicken and berries onto platter to keep warm. Add vinegar to pan, scrape browned bits free and boil on high heat until liquid is reduced by ⅓ and thicken. Pour sauce over chicken. Serves 2.

(Courtesy Valley View Blueberries.)

Crispy Hot and Tangy Thai Chicken

❖ ❖ ❖

4 cups Spectrum Naturals Pure Pressed Canola Oil *(or* Spectrum Naturals Super Canola Oil)
8 free-range chicken thighs
2 tablespoons tamari soy sauce
3 tablespoons Spectrum World Cuisine Thai Seasoning Oil
2 tablespoons garlic, finely minced
2 teaspoons ginger, finely minced
4 tablespoons Spectrum Naturals Organic Seasoned Brown Rice Vinegar
2 tablespoons cilantro, chopped
salt and fresh ground pepper to taste

Heat canola oil in a 4-quart saucepan to 350°. Meanwhile, wash and dry chicken pieces. In a mixing bowl, toss them in soy sauce, and reserve. Next, in a large sauté pan gently warm the Thai seasoning oil. Add garlic and ginger; gently cook for 1 minute. Add vinegar and continue to cook for 1 more minute. Remove from heat and reserve while you cook the chicken. Lower the chicken pieces into hot canola oil. Deep fry for 6 minutes, turning often. Remove chicken pieces and dry on paper towels for 2 minutes. Return the chicken to the hot oil for 4 minutes, turning often. Remove from oil and drain well. Meanwhile reheat garlic/ginger vinegar mixture. Toss cooked chicken in hot and tangy sauce and sprinkle with cilantro. Arrange well-coated chicken on a serving platter. Season with salt and pepper. Serve with salt and pepper. Serve hot or cold. Serves 4.

(Recipe created by Chef Gary Jenanyan.)

Grilled Marinated Chicken

❖ ❖ ❖

¼ cup Nakano Seasoned Red Wine Vinegar
1 pound skinless, boneless chicken breasts
black pepper and fine herbs

Pour vinegar over single layer of chicken. Sprinkle lightly with pepper and herbs. Refrigerate and marinate, covered, for at least 1 hour; drain. Grill chicken on one side 8–10 minutes or until light brown. Turn and baste with remaining marinade, then grill other side 6–8 minutes or until brown. Heat remaining marinade and pour over chicken. Serves 4.

Mediterranean Simmered Chicken

❖ ❖ ❖

2 pounds chicken, skinned (breasts and thighs)
1 (14½-ounce) can stewed tomatoes
1 (8-ounce) can tomato sauce
⅓ cup stuffed green olives
3 tablespoons Four Monks Red Wine Vinegar (Nakano)
1 tablespoon olive oil
1 teaspoon oregano, crushed
¼ teaspoon each salt and pepper
4 cloves garlic, chopped
3 small zucchini, sliced.

Cut chicken breasts in half across the bone. Combine chicken and remaining ingredients except zucchini in a large pot. Bring to a boil. Lower heat; cover and simmer 45 minutes. Add zucchini; cook an additional 5–7 minutes. Serve over hot cooked rice or pasta, if desired. Serves 4.

Polynesian Chicken

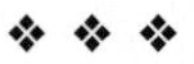

1 pound skinless boneless chicken breasts
1 medium green bell pepper, cut into 1-inch chunks
2 tablespoons butter or margarine
¼ teaspoon salt
dash pepper
2 cans (8 ounces each) pineapple chunks
½ cup water
⅓ cup Heinz Apple Cider Vinegar
2 tablespoons brown sugar
2 tablespoons soy sauce
1 teaspoon ginger
2½ tablespoons cornstarch
2½ tablespoons water
hot cooked rice
toasted slivered almonds

Cut chicken into strips about 2 inches long. In large skillet, sauté chicken and green pepper in butter just until chicken changes color. Season with salt and pepper. Stir in pineapple, pineapple liquid, and next 5 ingredients. Cover; simmer 10–12 minutes or until chicken is cooked. Combine cornstarch and 2½ tablespoons water; stir into chicken mixture. Cook until sauce is thickened, stirring constantly. Serve over rice; garnish with almonds. Makes 4 servings (about 4½ cups).

Seared Chicken Breast Stuffed with Spinach

4 boneless chicken breasts
4 tablespoons Mediterranean Spectrum Spread
24 spinach leaves, very coarsely chopped
salt and pepper
2 tablespoons Spectrum Naturals Super Canola Oil

Lay the chicken breasts flat on work surface. With a very sharp knife, create a pocket by cutting an incision horizontally through the middle of each breast, leaving it attached at one side. Spread 1 tablespoon of Mediterranean Spectrum Spread evenly into each breast. Stuff each breast with equal amounts of chopped spinach. Season with salt and pepper. Heat a nonstick pan over moderate heat. Add the canola oil. Cook the breasts over medium heat for approximately 4–5 minutes on each side or until the chicken is cooked and the spinach has wilted slightly. Remove from the pan and allow to rest for 3–5 minutes. Serves 4.

(Recipe created by Chef Gary Jenanyan.)

Sesame Chicken Sauté with Broccoli

❖ ❖ ❖

¼ *cup* Spectrum Naturals Pure Pressed Canola Oil *(or* Spectrum Naturals Super Canola Oil)
4 cups broccoli flowerets
¼ *cup* Spectrum Naturals Unrefined Toasted Sesame Oil
2 tablespoons tamari soy sauce
4 skinless, boneless, free-range chicken breasts, cubed
6 cloves garlic, finely minced
2 tablespoons Spectrum Naturals Organic Seasoned Brown Rice Vinegar
4 scallions, coarsely chopped
2 tablespoons sesame seeds
salt and ground pepper to taste

Heat the canola oil in a large skillet over medium heat. Add broccoli and sauté for 3 or 4 minutes, stirring constantly. Add sesame oil and soy sauce; continue to cook 1 more minute, stirring constantly. Add chicken and content to stir. Add garlic then vinegar. Continue to cook, stirring often until chicken is cooked through, 3 or 4 more minutes. Remove from heat, add scallions and sesame seeds. Season with salt and pepper. Serve immediately over rice or noodles. Serves 4.

(Recipe created by Chef Gary Jenanyan.)

Sweet and Sour Chicken

1½ cups Marsala wine
1 large onion, chopped fine
3 whole cloves
3 cloves garlic, chopped
1 large bay leaf
6 chicken breasts, 7 ounces each, skin on
flour seasoned with salt and pepper
3 ounces olive oil
10 ounces chicken broth
3 tablespoons sugar
6 ounces red or white wine vinegar
¼ cup raisins (optional)
¼ cup pine nuts (optional)

In a saucepan, heat the Marsala wine, onion, cloves, garlic, and bay leaf. Just before it comes to a boil, pour over the chicken breasts in a shallow glass baking dish. Cover and refrigerate overnight or for at least 6 hours. Remove breasts from marinade, dredge in seasoned flour, and sauté in large skillet for 3 or 4 minutes on each side. Set aside on a plate. Pour off any excess oil from skillet. After discarding cloves and bay leaf from marinade, add this liquid to the skillet. Simmer for 5 minutes, then return breasts to the skillet, spooning sauce over the breasts. Add broth, stir, cover, and cook for 15 minutes, turning once or more. While chicken is simmering, heat sugar in a small saucepan until it melts to an amber color. Carefully stir in vinegar and, if you wish, the raisins and pine nuts. Pour this mixture over the breasts 2 or 3 minutes before they are done. Serves 6.

(Recipe by Chef Salvatore J. Campagna.)

Tomato and Herb Chicken

❖ ❖ ❖

1 medium onion, sliced
2 cloves garlic, minced
1 teaspoon dried rosemary leaves
½ teaspoon dried basil leaves
½ teaspoon dried thyme leaves
2 tablespoons vegetable oil
1 (16-ounce) can tomatoes, drained, cut into bite-size pieces
¾ cup Heinz Tomato Ketchup
¼–⅓ cup Heinz Apple Cider Vinegar
1 tablespoon brown sugar
½ teaspoon salt
dash pepper
2½–3 pounds broiler-fryer pieces, skinned
cornstarch-water mixture
hot cooked noodles

In Dutch oven or large skillet, sauté onion, garlic, and herbs in oil until onion is tender-crisp. Stir in tomatoes and next 5 ingredients. Add chicken. Bring to a boil; reduce heat and simmer, covered, 45–50 minutes or until chicken is tender. Thicken sauce with cornstarch-water mixture. Serve chicken and sauce with noodles. Makes 5–6 servings (about 3 cups sauce).

Tangy Chicken and Herbs

1 medium onion, sliced
2 cloves garlic, minced
½ teaspoon dried rosemary leaves
½ teaspoon dried basil leaves
½ teaspoon dried thyme leaves
1 tablespoon vegetable oil
1 (16-ounce) can tomatoes, drained, cut into bite-sized pieces
½ cup Heinz Tomato Ketchup
¼ cup Heinz Apple Cider Vinegar
½ teaspoon salt
⅛ teaspoon pepper
2½ to 3 pounds broiler-fryer pieces, skinned
cornstarch-water mixture
hot cooked noodles

In a Dutch oven or large skillet, sauté onion, garlic, and herbs in oil until onion is just tender. Stir in tomatoes and next 4 ingredients. Add chicken. Bring to a boil; reduce heat and simmer, covered, 35–40 minutes or until chicken is tender, turning and basting occasionally.

Remove chicken. To thicken sauce, gradually stir in mixture of equal parts cornstarch and water, simmering until thickened. Serve chicken and sauce with noodles. Makes 5–6 servings (about 2½ cups of sauce).

Turkey Wraps

❖ ❖ ❖

½ cup lite or regular mayonnaise
2 tablespoons Nakano Seasoned Rice Vinegar with Red Pepper *or* Nakano Seasoned Rice Vinegar with Roasted Garlic
⅛ teaspoon cayenne pepper
⅛ teaspoon ground cumin
⅛ teaspoon salt
4 (8-inch) flour tortillas or seasoned whole wheat tortillas, warmed if desired
4 leaves red leaf or romaine lettuce
⅓ pound deli slice turkey breast or smoked turkey breast
¾ cup julienned jicama (optional)
⅓ cup julienned carrot
1 cup shredded Monterey Jack cheese
alfalfa sprouts (optional)

In a small bowl, combine mayonnaise, vinegar, cayenne pepper, cumin, and salt. Spread half of mayonnaise mixture over each tortilla; top with lettuce and turkey. Spread remaining mayonnaise mixture over turkey; top with jicama, carrots, cheese, and, if desired, sprouts. Fold bottom of tortilla over filling; roll up burrito-style. Serves 4.

Main Meat Dishes

Beef, pork, and liver. What do these foods have in common? Even though fat is their common thread, they're packed with protein that health-conscious Americans can feel good about eating.

Researchers in Australia pitted a vegetarian diet (that included milk and eggs) against an equal-fat diet containing lean meat. In result, both diets lowered blood pressure and cholesterol.[1]

Both cuts of meat contain plenty of animal protein, B vitamins for better immunity, and blood-building iron. And when you team meat recipes with garlic, onions, olive oil—and vinegar—it becomes a healthy, mouthwatering dish that is great for you!

Hearty Garlic Chili
Japapeño Pepper Jelly Barbequed Ribs
Mediterranean Beef Stew
Sauerbrauten
Sweet and Sour Meatballs
Tropical Glazed Ribs

Hearty Garlic Chili

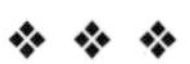

1½ pounds lean ground beef
6–8 cloves garlic, chopped
1 large onion, chopped
2 tablespoons chili powder
1 teaspoon oregano, crushed
1 teaspoon ground cumin
¼ cup Four Monks Red Wine Vinegar (Nakano)
2 (16-ounce) cans kidney beans, drained and rinsed
2 (8-ounce) cans tomato sauce
1 (12-ounce) jar hot or mild salsa

In a large pot, combine ground beef, garlic, onion, chili powder, oregano, and cumin. Cook on high until beef is cooked through. Add remaining ingredients. Lower heat; cover and simmer 45 minutes, stirring occasionally. For thicker chili, cook 10 minutes longer, uncovered. Serves 6–8.

Jalapeño Pepper Jelly Barbecued Ribs

❖ ❖ ❖

1 (10-ounce) jar Four Monks Mild Green, Tangy Red, *or* Hot Yellow Jalapeño Pepper Jelly
1 (15-ounce) can tomato sauce
2 tablespoons Four Monks Burgundy Cooking wine
2 tablespoons Four Monks Red Wine Vinegar (Nakano)
salt
4 pounds baby back ribs
pepper

Combine jelly, next 3 ingredients, and 1 teaspoon salt in saucepan. Simmer 15 minutes, stirring occasionally. Reserve. Cut ribs into two-rib serving pieces. Season well with salt and pepper. Place ribs on a rack in a shallow roasting pan. Roast at 450° for 30 minutes. Drain off fat. Reduce heat to 325°. Continue to roast, basting frequently with reserved sauce until a cut made near the center of a meaty section shows no pink, about 1 hour longer. Pour remaining sauce over ribs; serve. Makes 4–6 servings.

Mediterranean Beef Stew

❖ ❖ ❖

1 pound lean beef or *stew meat, cut into 1½-inch cubes*
2 tablespoons flour
2 tablespoons olive oil
1 medium onion, sliced
1 clove garlic, minced
1 (28-ounce) can crushed tomatoes, undrained
¾ cup canned beef broth
½ cup sliced pimento-stuffed green olives
⅓ cup dry red wine
¼ cup sundried tomatoes in oil, drained, thinly sliced
3 tablespoons Nakano Seasoned Rice Vinegar with Red Pepper *or* Nakano Seasoned Red Wine Vinegar—Italian Herb
1 tablespoon tomato paste
1 teaspoon salt, or to taste
¼ teaspoon freshly ground black pepper
¼ cup chopped fresh basil

Dredge meat in flour. Heat 1 tablespoon oil in a Dutch oven or large saucepan over medium heat until hot. Add half of meat; brown on all sides and transfer to a bowl. Repeat with remaining 1 tablespoon and meat. Add onions to Dutch oven; cook 5 minutes, stirring occasionally. Add garlic; cook 1 minute. Add remaining ingredients except basil. Return meat with any accumulated juices to Dutch oven. Bring to a boil. Reduce heat; cover and simmer 2 hours or until meat is tender. Stir in basil just before serving. Serves 4.

Sauerbraten

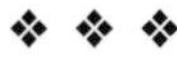

Marinade

1¼ cups dry red wine
1¼ cups red wine vinegar
2 quarts water
2 onions, sliced
8 black peppercorns, whole
10 juniper berries
3 bay leaves
2 cloves, whole

4 pounds beef bottom round
salt to taste
4 ounces vegetable oil
8 ounces onions, diced
4 ounces carrots, diced
4 ounces celery, diced
4 ounces tomato paste
2 ounces all-purpose flour
3 quarts beef broth
gingersnaps to taste

Combine all ingredients for the marinade and bring to a boil, then cool to room temperature. Remove all fat, gristle, and any membrane covering the meat. Season the beef round with salt and put it in the marinade. Refrigerate in a nonaluminum container for 3–5 days, turning 2 or 3 times daily. Remove meat from marinade. Strain and reserve marinade and reserve the onions and herbs separately. Bring the marinade to a boil (off center from heat) and skim off scum. Heat the oil in a braising pan, sear beef on all sides, remove, and reserve. Add diced vegetables and reserved onion-herb mixture. Brown lightly. Whisk in tomato paste then deglaze pan with reserved marinade and reduce this mixture by half. Sprinkle the flour into the reduced liquid and whisk thoroughly. Add the beef broth and whisk out any lumps. Bring to a simmer, place the beef round back in the braising pan, cover, and cook in a 300° oven until fork tender. Remove the meat and reduce the sauce. Remove any visible fat. Add the gingersnaps and cook sauce for 10 to 12 minutes or until the gingersnaps dissolve. Strain sauce through cheesecloth or very fine mesh strainer. Serve with potato pancakes and red cabbage for a traditional German dinner. Serves 10.

(Recipe created by Sal J. Campagna.)

Sweet And Sour Meatballs

❖ ❖ ❖

1 (8-ounce) can pineapple, crushed
½ cup Heinz Apple Cider Vinegar
¼ cup firmly packed brown sugar
2 tablespoons soy sauce
1 teaspoon ginger
1½ pounds lean ground beef
¾ cup dry bread crumbs
¼ cup milk
1 egg, slightly beaten
1 teaspoon salt
dash pepper
1 tablespoon vegetable oil
1 tablespoon cornstarch
1 tablespoon water

Drain pineapple, reserving liquid. Add water to reserved liquid to measure ¾ cup. Add vinegar and next 3 ingredients, set aside. Combine beef and next 5 ingredients lightly but well. Form into 30 meatballs, using a rounded tablespoon for each. Brown meatballs in oil in a large skillet; drain excess fat. Add pineapple liquid mixture. Cover; simmer 15–20 minutes or until meatballs are cooked, stirring occasionally. Stir in reserved pineapple. Combine cornstarch and water; stir into skillet. Cook until sauce is thick, stirring constantly. Makes 6 servings.

Tropical Glazed Ribs

3 1½ to 4 pound lean pork baby back ribs
¼ cup plus 2 tablespoons Nakano Seasoned Rice Vinegar–Original
¼ cup unsweetened pineapple juice or canned papaya nectar
¼ cup lite or regular soy sauce
1 tablespoon bottled or fresh minced ginger
1 teaspoon bottled or fresh garlic
3 tablespoons brown sugar
½ cup pineapple or peach preserves

Place ribs in a resealable plastic bag. Combine ¼ cup vinegar, pineapple juice, soy sauce, ginger and garlic; mix well. Pour over ribs. Close bag securely; turning to coat. Marinate in refrigerator at least 4 hours or up to 24 hours before cooking. Preheat oven to 375°. Drain ribs, reserving marinade. Place ribs, meaty side up on foil-lined shallow baking sheet or jelly roll pan. Bake 30 minutes. Turn; continue to bake 15 minutes. Combine ½ cup remaining marinade (discard any remaining marinade) and brown sugar in a small saucepan. Simmer uncovered until slightly thickened and reduced to ⅓ cup, about 5 minutes. Turn ribs meaty side up; brush with brown sugar mixture. Return to oven; bake 20–25 minutes or until ribs are browned and glazed. Cool 10 minutes. Meanwhile, combine remaining 2 tablespoons vinegar with preserves; mix well. Cut ribs into individual pieces. Serve warm or at room temperature with dipping sauce. 12 servings.

Desserts

Surprise! Sweet foods can be good for you! Our vinegar desserts contain plenty of healthy ingredients such as yogurt, melons, and raisins. These edibles are nutritious foods—and can cure a sugar craving, too. And don't forget. Vinegar coupled with these naturally sweet treats makes dessert a healing delight.

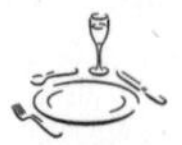

Low-Fat Peach and Yogurt Topping
Melon Sorbet
Old-Fashioned Raisin Pie
Strawberries with Orange and Balsamic Vinegar
Vinegar Pastry
Vinegar Pie

Low-Fat Peach and Vanilla Yogurt Topping

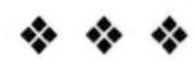

2 *cups low-fat plain yogurt*
4 *teaspoons pure vanilla extract*
6 *tablespoons pure maple syrup*
4 *tablespoons* Spectrum Naturals Organic Peach, Mango, *or* Raspberry Vinegars

Whisk together all ingredients in stainless steel or glass bowl. Combine with a chilled fresh fruit salad. For a variation, add chopped walnuts, sliced almonds, or toasted pecans. Makes 2½ cups.

Also makes an excellent:

- dip with fresh fruit spears
- accompaniment to granola or your favorite breakfast cereal
- garnish for waffles and pancakes
- topping on your favorite chocolate, spice, or pound cake

Melon Sorbet

❖ ❖ ❖

2 ripe sweet melons, halved and deseeded
½ cup icing sugar, sifted
6 tablespoons white wine vinegar
2 egg whites, large

Scoop flesh from melons and place in a food processor with sugar and vinegar. Blend to a puree. Place in a freezer-proof container; cover and freeze for 4–5 hours. Whisk egg whites until stiff, then blend with the mushy sorbet. Freeze until solid. Leave to stand at room temperature for 10–15 minutes before serving.

(The Vinegar Institute.)

Old-Fashioned Raisin Pie

❖ ❖ ❖

2 cups raisins
2 cups water
½ cup packed brown sugar
2 tablespoons cornstarch
½ teaspoon cinnamon
¼ teaspoon salt
1 tablespoon vinegar
1 tablespoon butter or margarine
pastry for double 9-inch crust

Combine raisins and water; boil 5 minutes. Blend sugar, cornstarch, cinnamon, and salt. Add to raisins and cook, stirring until clear. Remove from heat. Stir in vinegar and butter. Cool slightly. Turn into pastry-lined pan. Cover with top pastry or lattice strips. Bake at 425° about 30 minutes or until golden brown. Yield: One 9-inch pie

(Indian Summer, Inc.)

Strawberries with Orange and Balsamic Vinegar

❖ ❖ ❖

13 ounces fresh strawberries, (pint) washed, stemmed, sliced
½ cup fresh orange juice
1½–2 tablespoons balsamic vinegar
1 tablespoon fructose
6 sprigs fresh mint

Slice berries into medium-sized mixing bowl. Mix together orange juice, balsamic vinegar, and fructose. Pour over berries. Gently stir berries to cover liquid. Let sit for about 1 hour. Spoon into champagne glasses or other small decorative dishes. Garnish with sprig of mint. Serves 6.

(Recipe by Chef Michel Stroot of the Golden Door Spa.)

Vinegar Pastry

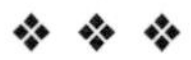

3 cups flour
1 cup shortening
½ teaspoon salt
1 egg
5 tablespoons cold water
1 tablespoon white vinegar
1 tablespoon water

Mix flour, shortening, and salt with a pastry blender until they become fine crumbs about the size of small peas. Beat egg with fork. Add cold water and vinegar. Combine liquid with flour and shortening mixture until thoroughly mixed. Divide dough into three balls of equal size. Each ball makes one single 9-inch pastry. Roll dough out and bake at 425° until lightly browned. (If wrapped well in plastic wrap, dough may be stored in refrigerator for approximately two weeks. Also freezes well. Remove from refrigerator several hours before rolling out.) Yield: Three single 9-inch pie shells.

(Source: Indian Summer, Inc.)

Vinegar Pie

4 eggs
1½ cups sugar
¼ cup butter or margarine, melted
1½ tablespoons cider or white vinegar
1 teaspoon vanilla extract
9-inch frozen pie shell, defrosted
chopped nuts (optional)
whipped cream (optional)

Preheat oven to 350. In a large mixing bowl, combine eggs, sugar, butter, vinegar, and vanilla; mix well. Pour into pie shell. Bake until firm, about 50 minutes. Cool on a rack. Serve garnished with chopped nuts or whipped cream, if desired. Yield: one 9-inch pie.

(Indian Summer, Inc.)

Before *You* Use Vinegar

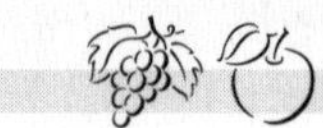

If you listen to the stories, each testimony of vinegar healing leads people to use it again and again. You, too, may experience the good of vinegar—inside or outside your body. If you acknowledge that an estimated 98 percent of Americans have vinegar already in their households, it just might be worth paying attention to.

The exciting old and new ingredients in potassium-plentiful *apple cider* and *now* antioxidant-rich *red wine vinegars* are enough to get you started. And don't forget the variety of health benefits that are provided by *rice, balsamic,* and *herbal vinegars,* too. Plus, these expert folk remedies and vinegar recipes (and some of my personal favorites) will keep you busy.

Keep in mind, however, if you want to prevent health ailments and lower your risk of disease (such as alcoholism *and* cancer, in my case), you have to learn the lessons of a healthy lifestyle (especially in the unpredictable twenty-first century) and practice them, too. Take the following steps:

1. Reduce the risk factor for diseases such as heart disease, stroke, and the most common forms of cancer by adopting a healthy diet, exercise, and stress-management program.

2. To combat some of the effects of air pollution and other environmental hazards, consider vitamin E and choosing foods rich in vitamin C, the vegetable form of vitamin A (beta-carotene), and a trace mineral called selenium.

3. Try to do a combination of aerobic exercise (walking, jogging, swimming, etc.), which is heart-healthy, and strength training (some type of weightlifting activity) for a minimum of three times a week, 20–30 minutes a day.

4. Forgo unhealthy vices and don't smoke; avoid certain foods, and alcohol.

5. And remember to stock your panty full of health-boosting vinegars, garlic, onions, olive oils—plenty of fresh fruits and vegetables—and enjoy a healthy diet!

PART 8

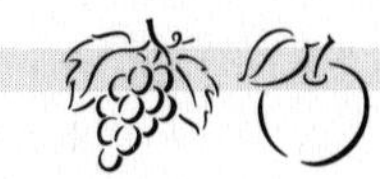

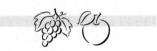

Vinegar Resources

Where Can You Buy Vinegar?

Vinegar in hand is better than Havla to come.
—Persian Proverb

As apple cider and red wine vinegars, and other types as well, continue to be touted for their powerful health benefits, quality vinegars for the health-conscious and specialty vinegars for vinegar lovers are popping up everywhere. Currently, a wide variety of vinegars can be bought in supermarkets and health food stores, as well as through mail-order and the Internet.

Here is a list of vinegars, from organic and natural to commercial brands. If you're interested in buying any of these vinegars and can't find them locally, just contact the manufacturers directly for the locations of stores nearest you.

VINEGARS PURCHASED IN RETAIL OUTLETS

Bertolli USA Inc.
300 Hamond Meadow Blvd.
Secaucus, NJ 07094-3621
201-863-2008

Balsamic Vinegars.

Boston Spice & Tea Co.
P.O. Box 38
Boston, VA 22713
877-966-4372

Boston Spice and Tea Company (founded in 1985) produces several herbal vinegars under the brand name O'Bannon's Mill Herbal Vinegars that utilize both red and white wine vinegars. They include:

- *Basil and Garlic:* used with pork or chicken (makes a great marinade), salads, and cooked greens. A great accompaniment to olive oil.
- *Old Thyme Herb Garden:* excellent with pork or chicken as a marinade and as a salad dressing used with olive oil.
- *Mediterranean Rose:* great marinade for lamb, pork, or chicken. Its mint, garlic, and rosemary adds an interesting flavor to fruit, rice, and pasta salads.

Bruno Pepper Co.
11291 North Ham Lane
Lodi, CA 95242
209-477-0066
Fax: 209-367-9311

Natural Red Wine Vinegar. Bruno provides a premium natural red wine vinegar made by using the "Orleans" method that is aged four full years in oak before it is released for sale. It is 75 grains in strength. A natural white wine vinegar is also available.

Bragg Live Foods
Box 7
Santa Barbara, CA 93102
www.bragg.com

Bragg Apple Cider Vinegar. This vinegar is organic, raw, and unfiltered with the "mother."

California Olive Oil Corp.
134 Canal Street
Salem, MA 01970
888-718-9830

Balsamic Vinegars.

Chicama Vineyards
Island of Martha's Vineyard
Stoney Hill Road
West Tisbury, MA 02575
508-693-0309

Wine Vinegars. Chicama make a wide variety of wine vinegars from their own wines, using the time-honored Orleans method.

Cypress Valley Gardens
P.O. Box 514
Wimberley, TX 78676-0514
512-847-5597

Gourmet Vinegars. Cypress Valley Gardens provides a potpourri of flavored vinegars such as strawberry, cranberry and herbal vinegars (garlic/chive, tarragon, basil/garlic, lemon/pepper, and balsamic).

Eden Foods, Inc.
701 Tecumseh Road
Clinton, MI 49236
800-248-0320

Apple Cider, Red Wine Vinegars, and *Specialty Vinegars.* Both apple cider and red wine vinegars are naturally fermented. Brown rice vinegar is sweet and smooth unlike most types of vinegar. Ume plum vinegar has a tart flavor derived from the organic acid in ume plums. Available in health food stores.

Gold Mine Natural Food Co.
7805 Arjons Drive
San Diego, CA 92126
1-800-475-3663

This organization is custom-tailored for those wanting macrobiotic and organic foods. They carry a wide variety of natural, organic vinegars: apple cider, which is naturally fermented, organic red wine, brown rice, ume, and rice malt.

Herb Patch Ltd.
471 South Street
Mail Address: Box 1111
Middletown Springs, VT 05757-1111
802-869-9333

Herbal and Fruit Vinegars.

Heinz USA
P.O. Box 57
Pittsburgh, PA 15230-0057
412-237-5757

Heinz U.S.A. has been established since 1885 and offers a variety of vinegars—apple cider, red wine, white distilled, garlic, wine, malt, salad, tarragon and balsamic. These types of vinegars are readily available in supermarkets.
Red Wine Vinegar—the most popular of specialty vinegars. Heinz begins with a specialty Burgundy wine which is manufactured from grapes grown in New York and Georgia. Its burgundy grapes give this vinegar a rich color and taste.
(See Part 7 for recipes using Heinz Vinegars.)

Live Food Products Inc.
Box 7
Santa Barbara, CA 93102-0007
805-968-1020

Apple Cider Vinegar. Live Foods Products offers organic apple cider vinegar.

Macrobiotic Company of America (M.C.O.A.)
799 Old Leicester Highway
Asheville, NC 28806
1-800-438-4730

Importers, distributors and processors of quality natural foods, including organic ume vinegar, organic brown rice vinegar, sweet brown rice vinegar, hato mugi vinegar, and organic yuzu vinegar—made from the juice of the rare Japanese citrus.

Maison Glass
111 East 58th Street
New York, NY 10022
212-755-3316/888-676-3663

Maison offers a domestic red wine vinegar and a special red wine raspberry vinegar, white wine vinegar with tarragon, and potato vinegar. Also, they have two Fini balsamic vinegars (one that is normally aged; the other 12 years aged) which are made in Italy.

Nakano Foods, Inc.
55 Euclid Ave.
Suite 300
Mount Prospect, IL 60056
1-800-323-4358

Brand names of Nakano vinegars include Four Monks, Barengo, and Indian Summer which provide a wide variety of vinegars including:

- *Red Wine Vinegar*—Barengo Gourmet Red Wine Vinegar. It is naturally fermented using the Orleans method. It also has a higher acid level (7.5) than most other wine vinegars.
- *Natural and Original Rice Vinegar*—Natural rice vinegar is a smooth replacement for wine, cider, or white distilled vinegars in your favorite recipes. The light and tangy flavor of Nakano's seasoned vinegars can add gusto to your favorite meal.
- *Balsamic Wine Vinegar*—is imported from the Modena region of Italy. Barengo is made in a time consuming process that begins with flavorful Trebbiano grapes.

(See Part 7 of this book for recipes using Nakano products.)

Oregon Spice Co.
1630 S.E.. Rhine
Phoenix, OR 97535-2845

Rice Wine Vinegar.

Organic Food Products, Inc.
7980 Soquel Drive
Mailing Address: P.O. Box 550
Aptos, CA 95001-0550
408-782-1133

Organic Vinegars.

Pompeian Red Wine Vinegar
4201 Polasky Highway
Baltimore, MD 21224
410-276-6900
1-800-638-1224

Red wine, red wine garlic, and balsamic vinegars shipped from the Mediterranean. Pompeian Red Wine Vinegar is aged in Spain for 15 years. (See Part 7 of this book for recipes using their products.)

Rubinelli, Inc.
5845 W. Thirty-first Street
Cicero, IL 60804
1-800-656-8884

Importers of Italian balsamic vinegar.

Nick Sciabica & Sons
2150 Yosemite Ave.
Modesto, CA 95354
1-800-551-9612

Sciabica specializes in cold-pressed olive oils using eight varieties of California olives. They also provide natural red wine vinegar as well as balsamic vinegar imported from Modena, Italy.

Spectrum Naturals, Inc.
133 Copeland Street
Petaluma, CA 94952
1-800-995-2705

Spectrum Naturals (founded in 1986) offers a variety of vinegars, including:

- *Apple Cider Vinegar*: organic, unfiltered.
- *Italian Balsamic Vinegar*: imported from Modena, Italy; aged four years in wooden casks; no artificial coloring.
- *Organic Italian Wine Vinegar*: imported from Modena, Italy; no added sulfites.
- *Organic Vinaigrettes*: dressings made with organic flax oil (rich in healthful omega-3 fatty acids), available in three flavors: balsamic, ginger-garlic and raspberry.

Spectrum Naturals also carries a full line of oils, including unrefined extra virgin olive oil and organic flax oils. Spectrum Organic Products offers a wide range of organic foods, including Millina's Healthy Kitchen organic pastas and pasta sauces with added omega-3 fatty acids. (See Part 7 of this book for recipes using Spectrum products.)

Tree of Life, Inc.
P.O. Box 410
1750 Tree Boulevard
St. Augustine, FL 32085
1-800-260-2424
www.treeoflife.com

Tree of Life is a major distributor to health food stores throughout the U.S. They have their own organic apple cider vinegar, raw and unfiltered, made exclusively from fresh whole organic Gravenstein apples, naturally processed to a mellow perfection.

Tree of Life also distributes Bragg apple cider vineger and all the Spectrum Naturals vinegars, as well as many other health food products which are also available in health food stores.

Valley View Blueberries
21717 N.E. 68th Street
Vancouver, WA 98682-9060
1-800-323-7743

Blueberry Gourmet Vinegar: contains white vinegar, red wine vinegar, blueberries and lemon juice. Certified pesticide-free. Blueberries are one of nature's best health and beauty aids. Research from Tuft's University has shown blueberries to contain age-defying and health-boosting antioxidants. Blueberries also contain vitamins A and C, iron, potassium and magnesium.

Valley View also markets dried blueberries which are certified pesticide-free, with no sugar or sulfites added. They also carry a blueberry fruit and nut mix, a unique blend of blueberries, cherries, cranberries, cashews, walnuts, hazelnuts and almonds. No salt, sugar, sulfites, or other preservatives.

Widow's Mite Co.
1309 P Street NW
Washington DC 20005
877-678-5754
http://www.widowsmitevinegar.com

Creole Spiced Vinegar: A unique vinegar, chock-full of herbs and spices, which tastes great on salads, seafood, poultry and other foods.

Vinegar Online

To save time and money, browsing the Internet for healthful vinegar is preferred by countless people. Not only do you get ingredient information on specific products, you can order easily right at home.

Bragg Live Foods
www.bragg.com

Bragg Apple Cider Vinegar. Organic, raw, unfiltered, with the "mother."

Dean & De Luca
HBergstein@corp.dean-deluca.com
Gourmet and specialty cider and flavored vinegars.

Hoosier Herbal Remedies
www.ezlinks.com/herbal
bnewsom@iquest.net

Grandma's Vim and Vigor, a Kentucky Mountain Recipe is an apple cider vinegar and herbal tonic.

Robert Rothchild's Gourmet
http://www.robertrothschild.com/VODRV.asp
Raspberry Vinegar

Information on Vinegar

The Vinegar Institute
Suite 500-D
5775 Peachtree-Dunwoody Road
Atlanta, GA 30342
404-252-3663
www.versatilevinegar.org
Contact: Linda Whitley

An age-old international trade association that represents vinegar manufacturers and bottlers in the United States, as well as producers in Australiz, Brazil, Canada, Germany, Italy, Japan, Panama, Sri Lanka, and South Korea. Companies manufacturing and/or bottling vinegar qualify for active membership in The Institute, and suppliers of goods or services to the vinegar industry are eligible suppliers. Their job is to make sure vinegar is labeled correctly, and they test on-the-market vinegars for authenticity to protect the consumer.

Vinegar Connoisseurs International
http://www.vinegarman.com

Lawrence Diggs is an international consultant to vinegar makers and author of *Vinegar*. He offers a wide variety of vinegar-related website links which are fun, fascinating, and informative.

Vinegar Connoisseurs International
P.O. Box 41
Roslyn, SD 57261
605-486-4536

A must-join organization for vinegar lovers. You'll enjoy a quarterly newsletter, discounts on selected vinegar products, introduction to exotic vinegars, and notices of stores with great vinegar sections and selections.

As of this writing, I find that more manufacturers and retail outlets could be added to this list. However, because of the popularity and varied types of vinegar to choose from, it is impossible to keep up with all the new companies marketing such products.

Notes

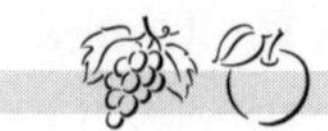

Chapter 1: The Power of Vinegar

1. Lawrence Diggs, *Vinegar* (Quiet Storm Trading Company, 1989), 249.
2. Jama, 1998:280:1569–1575.
3. D.C. Jarvis, *Folk Medicine: A New England Almanac of Natural Health Care from a Noted Vermont Country Doctor* (Fawcett Crest, 1958), 62.
4. Dr. Paul C. Bragg and Dr. Patricia Bragg, *Apple Cider Health System* (Health Science, 1995).
5. *Williams-Sonoma Essentials Vinegars*, ed. Chuck Williams (Weldon Owen Inc., 1994), 8.
6. Maggie Oster, *Herbal Vinegar* (Storey Communications, 1994), 6.

Chapter 2: A Genesis of Sour Wine

1. Lawrence Diggs, *Vinegar* (Quiet Storm Trading Company,1989), 249.
2. Op. cit., 214.
3. Ibid.

4. Emily Thacker, *The Vinegar Book* (Tresco Publishers, 1995), 4.
5. Maggie Oster, *Herbal Vinegar* (Storey Communications, 1994), 4.
6. Lawrence Diggs, *Vinegar* (Quiet Storm Trading Company, 1989), 39.
7.Ibid.
8.Maggie Oster, *Herbal Vinegar* (Storey Communications, 1994), 4.
9.Ibid.
10. Ibid.
11. Ibid.
12. Op. cit., 5.
13. Lawrence Diggs, *Vinegar* (Quiet Storm Trading Company, 1989), 214.
14. Op. cit., 214.
15. Maggie Oster, *Herbal Vinegar* (Storey Communications, 1994), 5.
16. Lawrence Diggs, *Vinegar* (Quiet Storm Trading Company, 1989), 23.
17. Op. cit., 27.

Chapter 3: A Historical Testimony

1. Lawrence Diggs, *Vinegar* (Quiet Storm Trading Company, 1989), 250.
2. Dr. Paul C. Bragg and Dr. Patricia Bragg, *Apple Cider Health System* (Health Science, 1995),11.
3. Ibid.
4. Ibid.
5. D.C. Jarvis, *Folk Medicine: A New England Almanac of Natural Health Care from a Noted Vermont Country Doctor* (Fawcett Crest,1958), 85.
6. Togo Kuroiwa, *Rice Vinegar: An Oriental Home Remedy* (Tokyo: Kenko Igakusha Co., 1977).
7. D.C. Jarvis, *Folk Medicine: A New England Almanac of Natural Health Care from a Noted Vermont Country Doctor* (Fawcett Crest,1958), 69.
8. Op. cit., 69.
9. Dr. Paul C. Bragg and Dr. Patricia Bragg, *Apple Cider Health System* (Health Science, 1995), 8.

10. Julian Whitaker, M.D., *Health & Healing* newsletter, May 1997 (Vol. 7, No. 5).
11. Ibid.
12. Ibid.
13. Ibid.
14. Ibid.

Chapter 4: Where Are the Secret Ingredients?

1. Dr. Paul C. Bragg and Dr. Patricia Bragg, *Apple Cider Health System* (Health Science, 1995), 1.
2. Product Data Sheet; Fleischmann's® *Apple Cider Vinegar*; Burns Philp Food Ingredients; June 15, 1998.
3. Maggie Oster, *Herbal Vinegar* (Storey Communications, 1994).
4. D.C. Jarvis, *Folk Medicine: A New England Almanac of Natural Health Care from a Noted Vermont Country Doctor* (Fawcett Crest, 1958), 68.
5. Dr. C. Bragg and Dr. Patricia Bragg, *Apple Cider Vinegar: Miracle Health System* (Health Science, 1995), 4.
6. Susan M. Lark, M.D., and James A. Richards, M.B.A., *The Chemistry of Success: Six Secrets of Performance* (Bay Books, 1999), 102.
7. Lawrence Diggs, *Vinegar and Health*, excerpted from "Vinegar"; VinegarAndHealth. html at www.vinegarman.com; 1

Chapter 5: Why Is Apple Cider Vinegar So Healthy?

1. Lawrence Diggs, *Vinegar* (Quiet Storm Trading Company, 1989), 248.
2. Editors of Prevention Magazine, *The Healing Foods Cookbook* (Rodale Press, 1991), 21.
3. Earl L. Mindell, R.Ph., Ph.D. with Larry M. Johns, *Amazing Apple Cider Vinegar: The Medicinal Miracle, plus the Curative, Cleaning and Cooking Virtues from Around the World* (Keats, 1996), 18.
4. *The Medical Post, Medical Bulletin*, Feb. 8, 1994.
5. *The Lancet*, March 1999.

CHAPTER 6: THE RED WINE VINEGAR CHRONICLE

1. Lawrence Diggs, *Vinegar* (Quiet Storm Trading Company, 1989), 250.
2. Togo Kuoiwa, *Rice Vinegar, An Oriental Home Remedy* (Tokyo: Kenko Igkusha Co., 1977), 6, 7.

CHAPTER 7: THE OLD AND NEW HEALTHFUL INGREDIENTS

1. Lawrence Diggs, *Vinegar* (Quiet Storm Trading Company, 1989), 250.
2. Product Data Sheet, Fleischmann's® Red Wine Vinegar, June 15, 1998.
3. M.C. Garcia-Parrilla, F.J. Heredia, and Ana M. Troncosco, *Phenolic Composition of Wine Vinegars Produced by Traditional Static Methods, Nahrung* 41 (1997, Nr. 4 S 232–235); M. C. Garcia-Parrilla, F.J. Heredia, Ana M. Troncoso, *The Influence of the Acetifiication Process on the Phenolic Composition of Wine Vinegars, Sciences DES* (1998, 211-221).
4. *Science*, 6/10/97; Harriet Brown, "*Cancer at the Millennium*," *Energy Times*, May 1999.

CHAPTER 8: TAPPING INTO THE FRENCH PARADOX

1. *France—The Good Life, Savored, Your Health*, April 18, 1995.
2. Allan Magaziner, D.O., *The Complete Idiot's Guide to Living Longer & Healthier* (Alpha Books, 1999), 56.
3. Robert Crayhon, M.S., *Robert Crayhon's Nutrition Made Simple*: A *Comprehensive Guide to the Latest Findings in Optimal Nutrition* (M. Evans and Company, 1994), 60.
4. Op. cit., 60-61.
5. Op. cit., 62.
6. Anne Schamberg, *Journal Sentinel Inc.*, Sun., May 7, 1995.

Chapter 9: Is Red Wine Good for You?

1. Lawrence Diggs, *Vinegar* (Quiet Storm Trading Company, 1989), 250.
2. American Heart Association Journal Report: "Weekly Consumption of Wine May Cut Stroke Risk"; *Stroke: Journal of the American Heart Association*, Dec. 1998.
3. Ibid.
4. Allan Magaziner, D.O., *The Complete Idiot's Guide to Living Longer & Healthier* (Alpha Books, 1999), 54.
5. Earl Mindell, R.Ph., Ph.D., *Earl Mindell's Supplement Bible* (Fireside, 1998); 134.
6. Allan Magaziner, D.O., *The Complete Idiot's Guide to Living Longer & Healthier* (Alpha Books, 1999), 54.

Chapter 10: Healthy Rice Vinegar

1. Togo Kuroiwa, *Rice Vinegar: An Oriental Home Remedy* (Tokyo: Kenko Igakusha Co., 1977), 179.
2. Based on Product Data Sheet Fleischmann's® Rice Vinegar, June 15, 1998.
3. Togo Kuroiwa, *Rice Vinegar: An Oriental Home Remedy* (Tokyo: Kenko Igakusha Co., 1977), 86.
4. Op cit.
5. Op. cit., 179.
6. Ibid.
7. Maggie Oster, *Herbal Vinegar* (Storey Communications, 1994), 12.
8. Togo Kuroiwa, *Rice Vinegar: An Oriental Home Remedy* (Tokyo: Kenko Igakusha Co., 1977), 159, 163.

Chapter 11: The Balsamic Vinegar Boom

1. Richard Simmons, "Ask Richard Simmons," *Woman's World*, June 6, 1995.

2. Bob Rubinelli, "All About Balsamic Vinegar," Oct. 11–12, 1995.
3. Based on Product Data Sheet Fleischmann's® Balsamic Vinegar, June 15, 1998.
4. Richard Simmons, "Ask Richard Simmons," *Woman's World*, June 6, 1995.

Chapter 12: Healing Herbal Vinegars

1. Lawrence Diggs, *Vinegar* (Quiet Storm Trading Company, 1989), 22.
2. Ray Sahelian, M.D., *Kava: The Miracle Antianxiety Herb* (St. Martin's Paperbacks, 1998), 164.
3. Daniel B. Mowrey, Ph.D., *Herbal Tonic Therapies* (Keats Publishing, 1993), 269.
4. Op. cit., 270.
5. Jim O'Brien, "The Oregano Prescription," *Your Health*, February 1998; 55.
6. Earl Mindell, R.Ph., Ph.D., *Earl Mindell's Supplemental Bible*, (Fireside, 1998), 115.
7. Op. cit., 135.
8. Laurel Dewey, "Don't Just Look at It!" *Your Health*, Dec. 10, 1996, 80.
9. *Journal of Neuroscience*; Research News Release by National Institutes of Health; Sept. 15, 1999.
10. A Modern Herbal Home Page, <//mgmh.html>; 1995 Electric Newt.

Chapter 13: Combining Vinegar and Garlic, Onion, and Olive Oil

1. Lawrence Diggs, *Vinegar* (Quiet Storm Trading Company, 1989), 250.
2. Dr. Arnold Pike, D.C. "Garlic's Natural Medicinal Qualities" *Let's Live* (Nov. 1990).
3. James O'Brien, *Garlic and Vinegar* (Globe, 1998), 30.

4. Robert Crayhon, *Nutrition Made Simple* (M. Evans and Company, Inc., 1994), 61.
5. Nancy G. Freeman, *Bring on the Olive Oil: The Mediterrean Diet, Get Up and Go!* February 1999, 10.
6. Op. cit., 9.
7. Ibid.
8. Ibid.
9. *Circulation: Journal of the American Heart Association* (1999; 99: 779–785).

Chapter 14: Vinegarmania: Hope or Hype?

1. Janice Cox, *Natural Beauty for All Seasons: 250 Simple Recipes and Gift-Giving Ideas for Year-Round Beauty*, (Henry Holt and Company, 1996), 55.

Chapter 15: Therapeutic Uses

1. D.C. Jarvis, *Folk Medicine: A New England Almanac of Natural Health Care from a Noted Vermont Country Doctor* (Fawcett Crest, 1958), 9.
2. Bonnie K. McMillen, *Connections Quarterly*, Summer 1998.
3. Ibid.
4. Ibid.
5. D.C. Jarvis, *Folk Medicine: A New England Almanac of Natural Health Care from a Noted Vermont Country Doctor* (Fawcett Crest, 1958), 182.
6. Bob Goldstein, *Love of Animals* (Dec. 1996), 6.
7. Douglas L. Langer, D.V.M., M.S., Veterinary Medical Teaching Hospital, University of California, Davis, "Enteroliths: Do We Have a Problem in California," 1992, 3.
8. D.C. Jarvis, *Folk Medicine: A New England Almanac of Natural Health Care from a Noted Vermont Country Doctor* (Fawcett Crest, 1958), 183.

Chapter 16: Vinegar Is Not for Everyone: Some Sour Views

1. William Shakespeare, *The Merchant of Venice* (Penguin U.S.A., 1989).
2. Susan M. Lark, M.D., and James A. Richards, M.B.A., *The Chemistry of Success: Six Secrets of Peak Performance* (Bay Books, 1999), 111.
3. Ibid.
4. Lawrence Diggs, "*Vinegar Cures a Lot of Things, But Not Everything*," excerpted from *The Vinegar Connoisseurs International Newsletter;* HealthNot Everything.html at www.vinegarman.com; 1.
5. Ibid.
6. Bill Evers, Ph.D., RD., and April Mason, Ph.D., *National Council Against Health Fraud Newsletter,* May/June1996, Vol. 19, No. 3; *FDA Consumer,* Jan.–Feb., 1996, pp.35–36.

Vinegar Recipes

1. The Editors of Prevention Magazine, *The Healing Foods Cookbook* (Rodale Press, 1991), 31.

About the Author

Cal Orey is an author and journalist. She has a master's in English (creative writing) from San Francisco State University and for the past decade has written hundreds of articles for a variety of national magazines. She specializes in topics on nutrition, human and pet health, beauty, and relationships. Her articles have appeared in publications such as *Woman's World, Woman's Day, Complete Woman, Men's Fitness, Your Health,* and *Let's Live.* She lives in Northern California.